Efficacy Analysis in Clinical Trials an Update

Ton J. Cleophas • Aeilko H. Zwinderman

Efficacy Analysis in Clinical Trials an Update

Efficacy Analysis in an Era of Machine Learning

Springer

Ton J. Cleophas
Albert Schweitzer Hospital
Department Medicine
Sliedrecht, The Netherlands

Aeilko H. Zwinderman
Dept. Biostatistics and Epidemiology
Academic Medical Center
Amsterdam, The Netherlands

Additional material to this book can be downloaded from http://extras.springer.com.

ISBN 978-3-030-19920-3 ISBN 978-3-030-19918-0 (eBook)
https://doi.org/10.1007/978-3-030-19918-0

This Springer imprint is published by the registered company Springer Nature Switzerland AG
The registered company address is: Gewerbestrasse 11, 6330 Cham, Switzerland

Preface

The title *Machine Learning in Medicine: A Complete Overview* from the same authors was published by Springer in 2014. It showed that machine learning is helpful for the analysis of observational clinical research and surveys. To date machine learning has been rarely applied for the analysis of clinical trials.

Clinical trials have been developed for efficacy assessment of new medical treatments. They are, traditionally, assessed with continuous variables, and analyzed with t-statistic or analysis of variance. These tests are unable to handle many variables but this is no drawback, because multiple variables tend to even out by the randomization process, and are not further taken into account in the analysis. In contrast, modern medical computer files often involve hundreds of variables like genes and other laboratory values, and computationally intensive methods are required.

Fortunately, with the advent of the computer, a novel type of data analysis has developed machine learning. Although, commonly, used in social sciences, marketing research, operational research, and, occasionally, observational research, like surveys, it is virtually unused in the analysis of controlled clinical trials. Machine learning is different from traditional data analysis, because, unlike means and standard deviations, it uses proximities and patterns of data, data recognitions, thresholding, and trafficking. It is more flexible than traditional statistical methods and can process big data and hundreds of variables.

The main objective of the current edition is to systematically assess, for the first time, whether machine learning technologies can be applied for efficacy analysis of controlled clinical trials and whether it provides advantages. For the purpose, traditional statistical methods will be tested against important machine learning technologies, like Bayesian networks, evolutionary operations, decision trees, and support vector machines.

In 20 chapters, with 300 pages, many data examples will be given, both real data and hypothesized data, and analyses will be presented step by step, which is suitable for study as a stand-alone and for self-assessment through data files at extras.

springer.com. The edition has been written by experienced professors in medical statistics at various European universities and was prepared for a nonmathematical readership of medical and health professionals and students.

Sliedrecht, The Netherlands Ton J. Cleophas
Amsterdam, The Netherlands Aeilko H. Zwinderman

Contents

Chapter 1
Traditional and Machine-Learning Methods for Efficacy Analysis

Contents

Abstract This chapter reviews the general principles of traditional efficacy analyses of clinical trials in a nonmathematical fashion. First, t-tests and analyses of variance, both paired and unpaired, are explained as methods for testing the significance of difference between a new and control treatment. Instead of treatment modalities as causal outcome factors, many more causal factors of health and sickness can be tested in clinical trials, like psychological, social, and physical factors. With non-Gaussian frequency distributions, rank testing is adequate, and various methods are reviewed. Regression analyses for adjustment of baseline covariates, and the discretization of continuous predictors for better data precision are explained. With discrete and discretized predictors three dimensional bar charts and chi-square tests

T. J. Cleophas, A. H. Zwinderman, *Efficacy Analysis in Clinical Trials an Update*,
https://doi.org/10.1007/978-3-030-19918-0_1

are appropriate. We live in an era of machine learning, and, also in this edition, traditional methods for efficacy analysis will be tested against machine learning methodologies. A summary of methodologies is given in this chapter.

Keywords Clinical trials · Traditional efficacy analysis · Machine learning for efficacy analysis

1.1 Introduction

Typical efficacy endpoints have their associated statistical techniques. For example, values of continuous measurements (e.g., blood pressures) require the following statistical techniques:

(a) if measurements are normally distributed: t-tests and associated confidence intervals to compare two mean values; analysis of variance (ANOVA) to compare three or more,
(b) if measurements have a non-normal distribution: Wilcoxon or Mann-Whitney tests with confidence intervals for medians.

Comparing proportions of responders or proportions of survivors or patients with no events involves binomial rather than normal distributions and requires a completely different approach. It requires a chi-square test, or a more complex technique otherwise closely related to the simple chi-square test, e.g., Mantel Haenszl summary chi-square test, logrank test, Cox proportional hazard test etc. Although in clinical trials, particularly phase III-IV trials, proportions of responders and proportion of survivors is increasingly an efficacy endpoint, in many other trials proportions are used mainly for the purpose of assessing safety endpoints, while continuous measurements are used for assessing the main endpoints, mostly efficacy endpoints. We will, therefore, focus on statistically testing continuous measurements in this chapter.

Statistical tests all have in common, that they try to estimate the probability that a difference in the data is true rather than due to chance. Usually statistical tests make use of a so-called **test statistic:**

Chi-square	for the chi-square test
t	for the t-test
Q_1	for nonparametric comparisons
Q	for nonparametric comparisons
q_1	for Newman-Keuls test
q	for Dunnett test
F	for analysis of variance
Rs	for Spearman rank correlation test.

These test statistics can adopt different sizes. Tables for t-, chi-square- and F-, Mann-Whitney-, and Wilcoxon-rank-sum-tests are published in most textbooks of statistics (see References). Such tables show us the larger the size of the test statistic, the more likely it is, that the null-hypothesis of no difference from zero or no difference between two samples is untrue, and that there is, thus, a true difference or true effect in the data. Most tests also have in common, that they are better sensitive or powerful to demonstrate such a true difference as the samples tested are large. So, the test statistic in most tables is adjusted for sample sizes. We say, that the sample size determines the degrees of freedom, a term closely related to the sample size.

1.2 The Principle of Testing Statistical Significance

The human brain excels in making hypotheses, but hypotheses may be untrue. When you were a child you thought that only girls could become a doctor, because your family doctor was a female. Later on, this hypothesis proved to be untrue. Hypotheses must be assessed with hard data. Statistical analyses of hard data starts with assumptions:

1. our study is representative for the entire population (if we repeat the trial, difference will be negligible.
2. All similar trials will have the same standard deviation (SD) or standard error of the mean (SEM).

Because biological processes are *full* of variations, statistics will give no certainties only chances. What chances? Chances that hypotheses are true/untrue. What hypotheses? E.g.:

(1) our mean effect is not different from a 0 effect,
(2) it is really different from a 0 effect,
(3) it is worse than a 0 effect.

Statistics is about estimating such chances/testing such hypotheses. Please note, that trials often calculate differences between a test treatment and a control treatment, and, subsequently, test whether this difference is larger than 0. A simple way to reduce a study of two groups of data, and, thus, two means to a single mean and single distribution of data, is, to take the difference between the two, and compare it with 0.

Data of a trial can be described in the form of a normal distribution graph with SEMs on the x-axis, and this method is adequate to test various statistical hypotheses. We will now focus on a very important hypothesis, the null-hypothesis. What it literally means is: no difference from a 0 effect: the mean value of our sample is not different from the value 0. We will try and make a graph of this null-hypothesis.

What does it look like in graph? H1 in the figure below is a graph based on the data of our trial with SEMs distant from mean on the x-axis (z-axis). H0 is the same graph with a mean value of 0 (mean ± SEM = 0 ± 1).

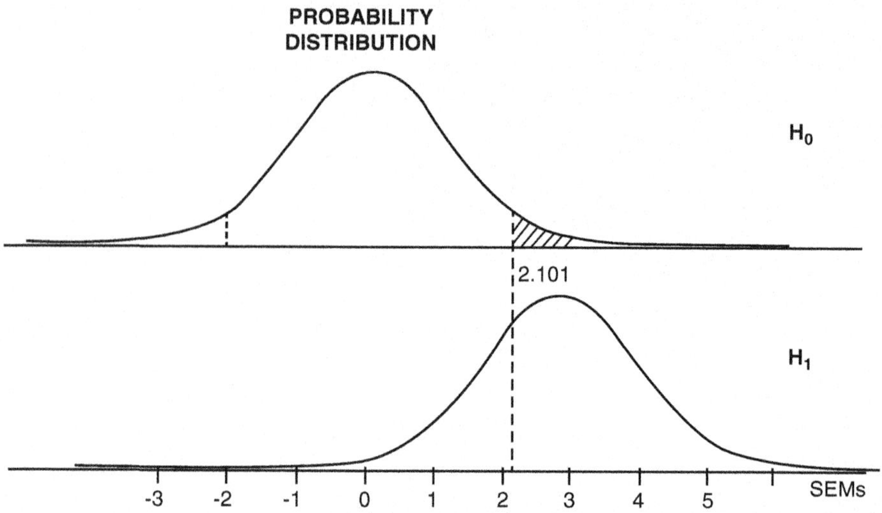

The above graph gives a null-hypothesis (H_0) and alternative hypothesis H_1 of an example of experimental data with sample size (n) = 20 and mean = 2.9 SEMs, and a t-distributed frequency distribution.

Now, we will make a giant leap from our data to the entire population, and we can do so, because our data are representative for the entire population. H1 is also the summary of the means of many trials similar to ours (if we repeat, differences will be small, and summary will look alike). H0 is also the summary of the means of many trials similar to ours, but with an overall effect of 0. Now our mean effect is not 0 but 2.9. Yet it could be an outlier of many studies with an overall effect of 0. So, we should think from now on of H0 as the distribution of the means of many trials with an overall effect of 0. If H0 is true, then the mean of our study will be part of H0. We cannot prove anything, but we can calculate the chance/probability of this possibility.

A mean value of 2.9 is far distant from 0. Suppose it belongs to H0. Only 5% of the H0 trials have their means > 2.1 SEMs distant from 0, because the area under the curve (AUC) > 2.1 distant from 0 is only 5% of total AUC. Thus, the chance that our mean belongs to H0 is <5%. This is a small chance, and we will reject this chance and conclude there is <5% chance to find this result. We, thus, reject the H0 of no difference from 0 at P<0.05. The AUC right from 2.101 (and left from −2.101 as will be soon explained) is called alpha = area of rejection of H0. Our result of 2.9 is far from 2.101. The probability of finding such a result may be a lot smaller than 5%. The underneath table shows the **t-table**, that can tell us exactly how small this chance truly is.

df	0.1	0.05	0.01	0.002
1	6.314	12.706	63.657	318.31
2	2.920	4.303	9.925	22.326
3	2.353	3.182	5.841	10.213
4	2.132	2.776	4.604	7.173
5	2.015	2.571	4.032	5.893
6	1.943	2.447	3.707	5.208
7	1.895	2.365	3.499	4.785
8	1.860	2.306	3.355	4.501
9	1.833	2.262	3.250	4.297
10	1.812	2.228	3.169	4.144
11	1.796	2.201	3.106	4.025
12	1.782	2.179	3.055	3.930
13	1.771	2.160	3.012	3.852
14	1.761	2.145	2.977	3.787
15	1.753	2.131	2.947	3.733
16	1.746	2.120	2.921	3.686
17	1.740	2.110	2.898	3.646
18	1.734	2.101	2.878	3.610
19	1.729	2.093	2.861	3.579
20	1.725	2.086	2.845	3.552
21	1.721	2.080	2.831	3.527
22	1.717	2.074	2.819	3.505
23	1.714	2.069	2.807	3.485
24	1.711	2.064	2.797	3.467
25	1.708	2.060	2.787	3.450
26	1.706	2.056	2.779	3.435
27	1.701	2.052	2.771	3.421
28	1.701	2.048	2.763	3.408
29	1.699	2.045	2.756	3.396
30	1.697	2.042	2.750	3.385
40	1.684	2.021	2.704	3.307
60	1.671	2.000	2.660	3.232
120	1.658	1.950	2.617	3.160
∞	1.645	1.960	2.576	3.090

The upper row gives the AUC-values right from trial results. Dfs means degrees of freedom. The 4 right-hand columns are trial results expressed in SEM-units distant from 0 (= **also t-values**). The left-hand column presents adjustment for numbers of patients (degrees of freedom (dfs), in our example two samples of 10 gives (20−2) = 18 dfs). AUC right from 2.9 means→ right from 2.878 means→ this AUC < 0.01. And so we conclude, that our probability not < 0.05, but even < 0.01.Note: the t-distribution is just an adjustment of the normal distribution, but a bit wider for small samples. With large samples it is identical to the normal distribution. For proportional data always the normal distribution is applied.

The t-table also gives two-tailed = two-sided AUC-values. This means, that the left and right end of the frequency distribution are tested simultaneously. A result > 2.101 here means both > 2.101 and < −2.101. If a result of + 2.101 was tested one sided, then the p-value would be 0.025 instead of 0.05.

1.3 The T-Value = A Standardized Mean Result of a Study

The t-table expresses the mean result of a study in SEM (standard error of the mean) – units. Why does it make sense to express mean results in SEM-units? Consider a cholesterol reducing compound, which reduces plasma cholesterol by 1.7 mmol/l ± 0.4 mmol/l (mean ± SEM). Is this reduction statistically significant? Unfortunately, there are no statistical tables for plasma cholesterol values. Neither are there tables for blood pressures, body weights, hemoglobin levels etc. The trick is to standardize your result.

$$\text{Mean} \pm \text{SEM} = \frac{\text{Mean}}{\text{SEM}} \pm \frac{\text{SEM}}{\text{SEM}} = \text{t-value} \pm 1$$

This gives us our test result in SEM-units with an SEM of 1. Suddenly, it becomes possible to analyze every study by using one and the same table, the famous t-table. How do we know, that our data follow a normal or t frequency distribution. For the purpose we have goodness of fit tests.

How was the t-table made? It was made in an era without pocket calculators, and it was hard work. Try and calculate in three digits the square root of the number 5. The result is between 2 and 3. The final digits are found by a technique called "tightening the data". The result is larger than 2.1, smaller than 2.9. Also larger than 2.2, smaller than 2.8, etc. It will take more than a few minutes to find out the closest estimate of $\sqrt{5}$ in three digits. This example highlights the hard work done by the U.S. Government's Work Project Administration by hundreds of women during the economic depression in the 1930s.

1.4 Unpaired T-Test

So far, we assessed a single mean versus 0, now we will assess two means versus each other. For example, a parallel-group study of two groups tests the effect of two beta-blockers on cardiac output.

	Mean ± SD			$SEM^2 = SD^2 / n$
group 1 (n =10)	5.9	± 2.4	liter / min	5.76 / 10
group 2 (n =10)	4.5	± 1.7	liter / min	2.89 / 10

Calculate: $mean_1 - mean_2$ = mean difference =1.4
Then calculate pooled $SEM = \sqrt{SEM_1{}^2 + SEM_2{}^2} = 0.930$

Note: for SEM of difference: take the square root of the sums of squares of separate SEMs, and, so, reduce analysis of two means and two SEMS to one mean and one SEM. The significance of difference between two unpaired samples of continuous data is assessed by the formula:

$$\text{mean}_1 - \text{mean}_2 \pm \sqrt{\text{SEM}_1^2 + \text{SEM}_2^2} = \text{mean difference} \pm \text{pooled SEM}$$

This formula presents again a t-distribution with a new mean and a new SEM, i.e., the mean difference and the pooled SEM. The wider this new mean is distant from zero and the smaller its SEM is, the more likely we are able to demonstrate a true effect or true difference from no effect. The size of the test statistic is calculated as follows.

$$\text{The size of t} = \frac{\text{mean difference}}{\text{pooled SEM}} = 1.4/0.930 = 1.505$$

With $n = 20$, and two groups we have $20-2 = 18$ degrees of freedom. The t-table shows that a t-value of 1.505 provides a chance of > 5% that the null hypothesis of no effect can be rejected. The null-hypothesis cannot be rejected.

Note: If the standard deviations are very different in size, e.g., if one is twice the other, then a more adequate calculation of the pooled standard error is as follows.

$$\text{Pooled SEM} = \sqrt{\frac{(n_1 - 1)SD_1^2 + (n_2 - 1)SD_2^2}{n_1 + n_2 - 2} \times \left(\frac{1}{n_1} + \frac{1}{n_2}\right)}$$

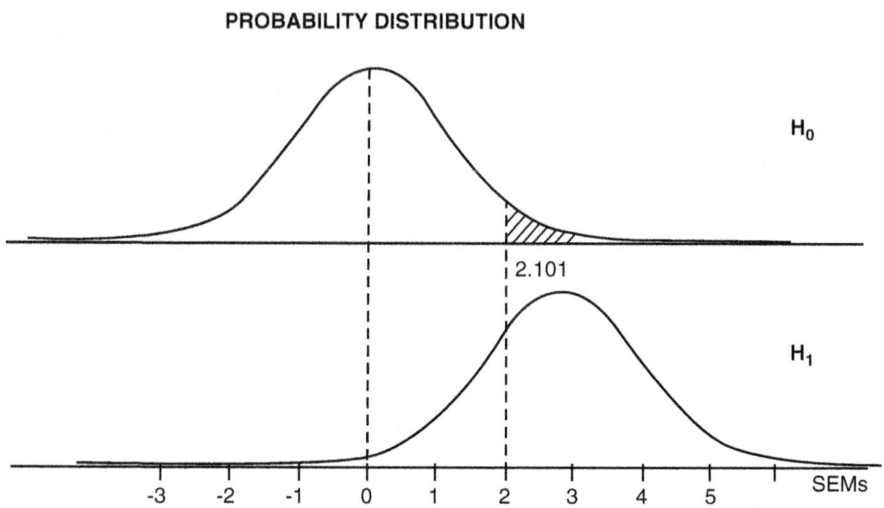

The above figure shows two t- distributions with n = 20: the lower curve gives H1 or actual SEM-distribution of the data, the upper curve gives H0 or null hypothesis of the study.

The lower graph of the above figure is the probability distribution of this t-distribution. H0 (the upper graph) is an identical distribution with mean = 0 instead of mean. Mean means here $\text{mean}_1 - \text{mean}_2$ and SEM is identical to the SEM of H1, and is taken as the null- hypothesis in this particular approach. With n = 20 (18 degrees of freedom) we can accept that 95% of all t-distributions with no significant treatment difference from zero must have their means between −2.101 and +2.101 SEMs distant from zero. The chance of finding a mean value of 2.101 SEMs or more distant from 0 to 5% or less (we say $\alpha = 0.05$, where α is the chance of erroneously rejecting the null hypothesis of no effect). This means that we can reject the null-hypothesis of no difference at a probability (P) = 0.05. We have 5% chance of coming to this result, if there were no difference between the two samples. This is pretty small. We, therefore, conclude, that there is a true difference between the effects on cardiac output of the two compounds.

Also the F- and chi-square test will reject, similarly to the t-test, the null-hypothesis of no treatment effect, if the value of the test statistic is larger than would occur in 95% of the cases if the treatment had no effect. At this point we should emphasize, that, when the test statistic is not big enough to reject the null-hypothesis of no treatment effect, investigators often report no statistically significant difference, and discuss their results in terms of documented proof, that the treatment had no effect. All they really did, was, fail to demonstrate, that it did have an effect. The distinction between positively demonstrating, that a treatment had no effect, and failing to demonstrate, that it does have an effect, is subtle but very important, especially with respect to the small numbers of subjects usually enrolled in a trial. A study of treatments, that involves only a few subjects, and then fails to reject the null-hypothesis of no treatment effect, may arrive at that conclusion, because the statistical procedure lacked power to detect the effect because of a too small sample size, even though the treatment did have an effect.

1.5 Null-Hypothesis Testing of Three or More Unpaired Samples

If more than two samples are compared, things soon get really complicated, and the unpaired t-test can no longer be applied. Usually, statistical software, e.g., SAS or SPSS Statistical Software, will be used to produce F- or P-values, but the table underneath gives a brief summary of the principles of multiple groups analysis of variance (ANOVA) applied for this purpose. With ANOVA the outcome variable (Hb, hemoglobin-level in the example) is often called the dependent variable, while the groups-variable is called the independent factor (SPSS commands are: Compare means; one-way ANOVA). If additional groups-variables are in the data (gender, age classes, comorbidities), then SPSS will require using the General Linear Model (univariate).

Unpaired ANOVA 3 groups

Total variation

Between group variation | within group variation

In ANOVA:

Variations are expressed as sums of squares (SS), and can be added up to obtain total variation. Assess, whether between-group variation is large compared to within-group variation.

Group	n patients	mean	SD
1	-	-	-
2	-	-	-
3	-	-	-

Grand mean = (mean 1 + 2 +3)/3

$SS_{between\ groups} = n\ (mean_1 - grand\ mean)^2 + n\ (mean_2 - grand\ mean)^2 + \ldots.$

$SS_{within\ groups} = (n\text{-}1)\ SD_1^{\ 2} + (n\text{-}1)\ SD_2^{\ 2} + \ldots..$

$$F = \frac{SS\ between\ groups\ /dfs}{SS\ within\ groups\ /\ dfs} = MS_{between} / MS_{within}$$

F-table gives P-value

Effect of 3 compounds on Hb

Group	n patients	mean	SD
1	16	8.7125	0.8445
2	16	10.6300	1.2841
3	16	12.3000	0.9419

Grand mean = (mean 1 + 2 +3)/3 = 10.4926

$SS_{between\ groups} = 16\ (8.7125\text{-}10.4926)^2 + 16\ (10.6300 - 10.4926)^2 + \ldots.$

$SS_{within\ groups} = 15 \times 0.8445^2 + 15 \times 1.2841^2 + \ldots\ldots..$

F = 49.9 and so P <0.001

Note: In case of 2 groups: ANOVA = unpaired T-test ($F=T^2$). Dfs means degrees of freedom, and equals 3n - 3 for SS_{within}, and (3-1) = 2 for $SS_{between}$.

1.6 Three Methods to Test Statistically a Paired Sample

The underneath table gives an example of a placebo-controlled clinical trial to test efficacy of a sleeping drug.

	hours of sleep				
patient	drug	placebo	difference	mean	SS
1	6.1	5.2	0.9	5.7	0.53
2	7.0	7.9	-0.9	7.5	
3	8.2	3.9	4.3		
4	7.6	4.7	2.9		
5	6.5	5.3	1.2		
6	7.8	5.4	3.0		
7	6.9	4.2	2.7		
8	6.7	6.1	0.6		
9	7.4	3.8	3.6		
10	5.8	6.3	-0.5		
Mean	7.06	5.28	1.78		
SD	0.76	1.26	1.77		
grand mean	6.17				

First Method
First method is simply calculating the SD of the mean difference d by looking at the column of differences (d-values) and using the standard formula for variance between data

$$\text{SD paired differences} = \sqrt{\frac{\sum (d - \bar{d})^2}{n - 1}} = 1.79$$

Next we find SEM of the mean difference by taking SD/$\sqrt{n} = 0.56$
Mean difference $\pm$ SEM $= 1.78 \pm 0.56$
Similarly to the above unpaired t-test we now can test the null hypothesis of no difference by calculating

$$\begin{aligned} t &= \frac{\text{Mean difference}}{\text{SEM}} = 1.78/0.56 \\ &= 3.18 \text{ with a sample of 10 (degrees of freedom} = 10 - 1) \end{aligned}$$

The t-table shows that $P < 0.02$. We will have <2% chance to find this result, if there were no difference, and accept, that this is sufficient to assume, that there is a true difference.

Second Method
Instead of taking the column of differences we can take the other two columns, and use the underneath formula for calculating the SD of the paired differences

$$= SD_{\text{paired difference}}$$
$$= \sqrt{\left(SD_1^2 + SD_2^2 - 2r \cdot SD_1 \cdot SD_2\right)}$$
$$= \sqrt{\left(0.76^2 + 1.26^2 - 2r \cdot 0.76_1 \cdot 1.26\right)}$$

R (or r) is the Pearson correlation coefficient. As r can be calculated to be + 0.26, we can now conclude that

$$SD_{\text{paired differnce}} = 1.79$$

The remainder of the calculations is as above.

Third Method

The third method is the F test using analysis of variance (ANOVA). We have to calculate SS (sum of squares) e.g., for the above table:

The third method is the F test using analysis of variance (ANOVA). We have to calculate SS (sum of squares) e.g., for the above table:

$SS_{\text{within subject 1}} = (6.1-5.7)^2 + (5.2-5.7)^2 + \ldots.. = 0.53$
grand mean $(7.06+5.28)/2 = 6.17$
$SS_{\text{within subject}} = SS_{\text{within subject1}} + SS_{\text{within subject2}} + SS_{\text{within subject3}} + \ldots.$
$SS_{\text{treatment}} = (7.06-6.17)^2+(5.28-6.17)^2$

$SS_{\text{residual}} = SS_{\text{within subject}} - SS_{\text{treatment}}$

An ANOVA table of these data is below.

Source of variation	Sum of Squares (SS)	degrees of freedom (dfs)	mean square MS=SS/dfs)	F = MS treatment / MS residual
between subjects		2 (m)		
within subjects		10 (n x (m-1))		
treatments		1 (m-1)		$F = 10.11, p < 0.02$
residual		9 (n-1)		
total		22		

The ANOVA table shows the procedure. Note m is number of treatments, n is number of patients. The ANOVA is valid not only for two repeated measures but also for multiple repeated measures. For 2 repeated measures it is actually equal to the paired t-test (= first method). The results of the analysis of the two tests are similar, with F being equal to t^2.

Similarly, for unpaired samples, with two samples the one way ANOVA is equal to the unpaired t-test, but one-way ANOVA can also be used for multiple unpaired samples.

The above data can also be presented in the form of a linear regression graph.

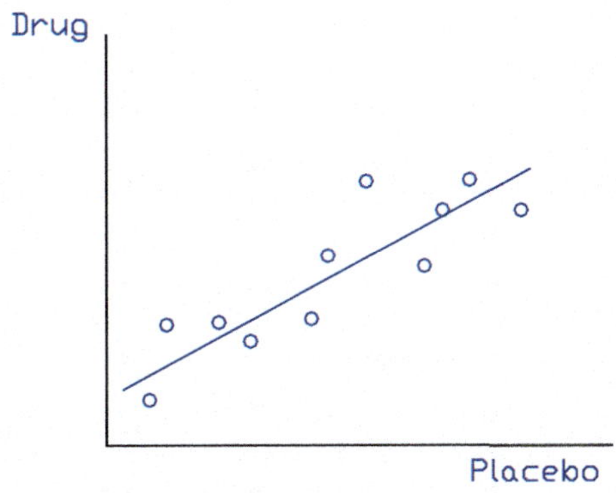

The above figure shows paired data laid out in the form of a linear regression.

$$y = a + b\,x\ (\text{effect drug}) = a + b\ (\text{effect placebo})$$

which can be assessed in the form of ANOVA:

$$F = r^2 = \frac{\text{regression sum of squares}}{\text{total sum of squares}}$$
$$= \frac{\left(\sum (x-\bar{x})(y-\bar{y})\right)^2}{\sum (x-\bar{x})^2 \sum (y-\bar{y})^2} = \frac{SP^2\ x \cdot y - \text{values}}{SS\ x\text{-values} \cdot SS\ y\text{-values}}$$

SS regression = SP^2 x. y –values / SS x -values
SS total = SS y
SS regression / SS total = r^2
SP indicates sum of products.

The underneath table gives an ANOVA table for the linear regression between paired samples.

Source of variation	Sum of Squares (SS)	degrees of freedom (dfs)	mean square MS=SS/dfs	F = MS regression / MS total
regression between samples	1.017	1	1.017	0.61, $P > 0.05$
residual	14.027	8	1.753	
total	15.044	9	1.672	

The above ANOVA table gives an alternative interpretation of the correlation coefficient; the square of the correlation coefficient, r, equals the regression sum of squares divided by the total sum of squares ($0.26^2 = 0.0676 = 1.017/15.044$) and, thus, is the proportion of the total variation that has been explained by the regression. We can say that the variances in the drug data are only for 6.76% determined by the variances in the placebo data, and that they are for 93.24% independent of the placebo data. With strong positive correlations, e.g., close to +1 the formula for SD and thus SEM reduces to a very small size (because $[SD_1^2 + SD_2^2 - 2\ r\ SD_1.SD_2]$ will be close to zero), and the paired t-test produces huge sizes of t, and, thus, huge sensitivity of testing. The above approach cannot be used for estimating significance of differences between two paired samples. And the method in the presented form is not very relevant. It will start, however, to be relevant, if we are interested in the dependency of a particular outcome variable upon several factors. E. g., the effect of a drug is better than placebo, but this effect still gets better with increased age. This concept can be represented by a multiple regression equation

$$y = a + b_1 x_1 + b_2 x_2$$

which in this example is

$$\text{drug response} = a + b_1.(\text{placebo response}) + b_2.(\text{age})$$

Although it is no longer easy to visualize the regression, the principles involved are the same as with linear regression.

1.7 Null-Hypothesis Testing of Three or More Paired Samples

If more than two paired samples are compared, things soon get really complicated, and the paired t-test can no longer be applied. Usually, statistical software (SAS, SPSS, R) will be used to produce F- and P-values, but the table gives a brief summary of the principles of ANOVA for multiple paired observations, used for this purpose.

The table below shows a repeated measurements ANOVA

Paired ANOVA 3 treatments in single group

Total variation
- Between subject variation
- Within-subject variation
  - Between treatment variation
  - Residual variation

Variations expressed as sums of squares (SS) and can be added up
Assess whether between treatment variation is large compared to residual variation.

Subject	treatment 1	treatment 2	treatment 3	SD^2
1	-	-	-	-
2	-	-	-	-
3	-	-	-	-
4	-	-	-	-
Treatment mean	-	-	-	

Grand mean = (treatment mean 1 + 2 + 3)/ 3 = ...

$SS_{\text{within subject}} = SD_1^2+SD_2^2+SD_3^2+..$
$SS_{\text{treatment}} = (\text{treatment mean } 1 - \text{grand mean})^2 + (\text{treatment mean } 2- \text{grand mean})^2 + ...$
$SS_{\text{residual}} = SS_{\text{within subject}} - SS_{\text{treatment}}$

$$F = \frac{SS_{\text{treatment}}/\text{dfs}}{SS_{\text{residual}}/\text{dfs}}$$

F table gives P-value.

Effect of 3 treatments on vascular resistance (blood pressure / cardiac output).

Person	treatment 1	treatment 2	treatment 3	SD^2
1	22.2	5.4	10.6	147.95
2	17.0	6.3	6.2	77.05
3	14.1	8.5	9.3	18.35
4	17.0	10.7	12.3	21.4
Treatment mean	17.58	7.73	9.60	

Grand mean = 11.63

$SS_{\text{within subj}} = 147.95 + 77.05 + ...$
$SS_{\text{treatment}} = (17.58 - 11.63)^2 + (7.73 - 11.63)^2 + ...$
$SS_{\text{residual}} = SS_{\text{within subject}} - SS_{\text{treatment}}$

$F = 18.2$ and so $P < 0.025$

Note: in case of 2 treatments: repeated measurements-ANOVA produces the same result as the paired t-test ($F = t^2$), dfs = degrees of freedom equals (3-1) = 2 for $SS_{\text{treatment}}$, and (4-1) = 3 for SS_{residual}.

1.8 Null Hypothesis Testing with Complex Data

ANOVA is briefly addressed in the above Sects. 1.6 and 1.7. It is a powerful method for the analysis of complex data. ANOVA compares mean values of multiple cells, and can be classified in several manners: (1) one-way or two-way (left example gives one-way ANOVA with 3 cells, right example two-way ANOVA with 6 cells), (2) unpaired or paired data, if the cells contain either non-repeated or repeated data (otherwise called repeated measures ANOVA), (3) data with or without replication, if the cells contain either multiple data or a single datum, (4) balanced or unbalanced, if the cells contains equal or differing numbers of data.

The Table below shows, that ANOVA compares multiple cells with means, and can be classified several ways.

(1) One-way		Two-way			
mean bloodpressure		mean results of treatments 1-3			
group 1	..... (SD...)		1	2	3
		males	....	.....	.....
group 2	......				
group 3	.....	females	.....	......	.....
(2) unpaired data		unpaired data / paired data			
(3) with replication		with replication / without replication			
(4) balanced / unbalanced		balanced / unbalanced			

Sometimes samples consist of data that are partly repeated, and partly non-repeated. E.g., 10 patients measured 10 times produces a sample of $n = 100$. It is not appropriate to include this sample in an ANOVA-model as either entirely repeated or non-repeated. It may be practical, then, to use the means per patient as a summary measure without accounting its standard deviation, and perform simple tests using the summary measures per patient only. Generally, the simpler the statistical test the more statistical power.

1.9 Paired Data with a Negative Correlation

Not only crossover, but also parallel-group studies often include an element of self-controlling. E.g., observations before, during, and after treatment are frequently used as the main control on experimental variation. Such repeated measures will, generally, have a positive correlation: those who respond well during the first observation are more likely to do so in the second. This is, however, not necessarily so. When drugs of completely different classes are compared, patients may fall apart into different populations: those who respond better to one and those who respond better to the other drug. For example, patients with angina pectoris, hypertension, arrhythmias, chronic obstructive pulmonary disease, unresponsive to one class of drugs, may respond very well to a different class of drugs. This situation gives rise to a negative correlation in a paired comparison. Other examples of negative correlations between paired observations include the following. A negative correlation between subsequent observations in one subject may occur, because fast-responders are more likely to stop responding earlier. A negative correlation may exist in the patient characteristics of a trial, e.g., between age and vital lung capacity, and in outcome variables of a trial, e.g., between severity of heart attack and ejection fraction. Negative correlations in a paired comparison reduce the sensitivity not only of studies testing differences but also of studies testing equivalences.

1.9.1 Studies Testing Significance of Differences

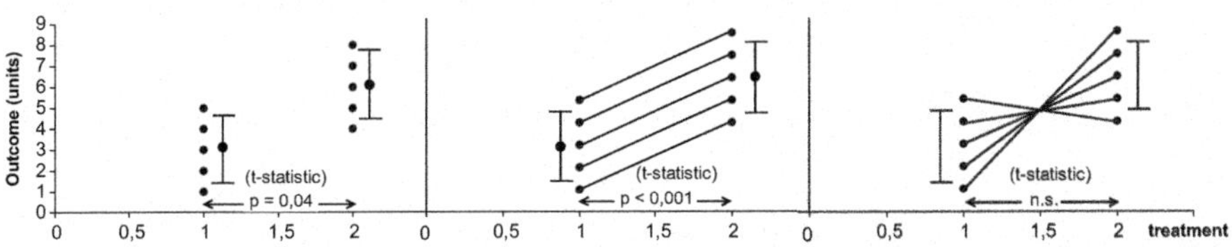

The above figure gives a hypothesized example of three studies: the left graph shows a parallel-group study of 10 patients, the middle and right graph show self-controlled studies of 5 patients each tested twice. T-statistics is employed according to the formula

$$t = \frac{\bar{d}}{SE}$$

Where $\bar{d}$ is the mean difference between the two sets of data (6−3 = 3) and the standard error (SE) of this difference is calculated for the left graph data according to

$$\sqrt{\frac{SD_1^2}{n_1} + \frac{SD_2^2}{n_2}} = 0.99$$

$SD_1$and SD_2 are standard deviations and n_1 and n_2 are numbers of observations in each of the groups. We assume that $n_1 = n_2 = n$.

$$t = 3/0.99 = 3.0$$

With 10 observations we can reject the null-hypothesis at p = 0.04.

With a positively paired comparison (middle graph) we have even more sensitivity. SE is calculated slightly different

$$SE = \frac{\sqrt{\sum (d\text{-}\bar{d})^2/(n-1)}}{\sqrt{n}} = 0$$

where d is the observed change in each individual and $\bar{d}$ is its mean.

$$t = \bar{d}/SE = 3/0 = \infty$$

with n = 5 we can reject the null-hypothesis at p < 0.001.

The right graph gives the negative correlation situation. SE calculated similarly to the middle graph data is 1.58, which means that

$$t = 3/1.58 = 1.89$$

The null-hypothesis of no difference cannot be rejected. Differences are not significant (n.s.).

When more than 2 treatments are given to one sample of patients, t-statistics is not appropriate and should be replaced with analysis of variance.

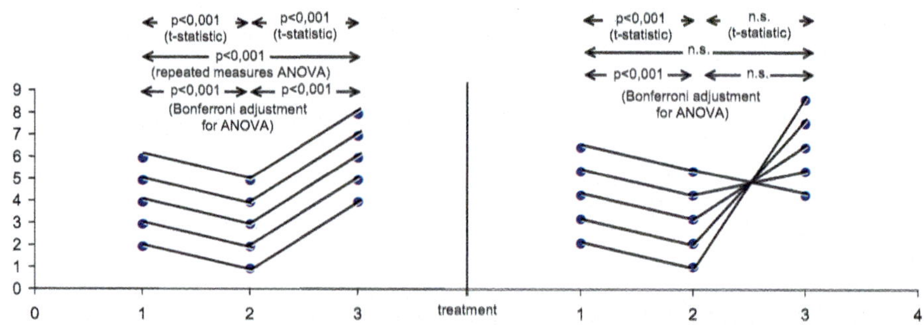

The above figure gives a hypothesized example of two studies where 5 patients are tested three times. Due to negative correlation between treatment 2 and 3 in the right graph study, the statistical significance test is negative unlike the left graph study, despite the identical mean results. In the left graph the correlation between treatment responses is positive, whereas in the right graph the correlation between treatment no. 3 and no. 2 is strong negative rather than positive. For the left graph data repeated measures analysis of variance (ANOVA) is performed.

The sum of squares (SS) of the different treatments is calculated according to

Patient	treatment 1	treatment 2	treatment 3	Mean	SD^2
1	6	5	8	6.3	4.67
2	5	4	7	5.3	4.67
3	4	3	6	4.3	4.67
4	3	2	5	3.3	4.67
5	2	1	4	2.3	4.67
Treatment mean	4	3	6		

Grand mean 4.3

$SS_{\text{within subjects}} = 4.67 + 4.67 + \ldots = 23.3$

$SS_{\text{treatments}} = 5\,[(4\text{-}4.3)^2 + (3\text{-}4.3)^2 + (6\text{-}4.3)^2] = 23.35$

$SS_{\text{residual}} = SS_{\text{within subjects}} - SS_{\text{treatments}} = 0$

Table 8. ANOVA table of the data

Source of variation	SS	dfs	MS
Within subjects	23.35	10	
Treatments	23.35	2	11.68
Residual	0	8	0

$$F = \frac{MS_{\text{treatments}}}{MS_{\text{residual}}} = \infty \qquad p < 0.001$$

This analysis permits concluding that at least one of the treatments produces a change. To isolate which one, we need to use a multiple-comparisons procedure, e.g., the modified Bonferroni t-test for ANOVA where

"$SE^2 = \Sigma(d-\bar{d})^2/(n-1)$" is replaced with "$MS_{\text{residual}}$". So, to compare, e.g., treatment no. 2 with treatment no. 3

$$t = \frac{6-3}{\sqrt{(MS_{\text{residual}})/n}} = \infty \quad p < 0.001$$

Of the right graph a similar analysis is performed.

Patients	treatment 1	treatment 2	treatment 3	Mean	SD^2
1	6	5	4	5.0	1.0
2	5	4	5	4.7	0.67
3	4	3	6	4.3	4.67
4	3	2	7	4.0	14.0
5	2	1	8	3.7	28.49
Treatment mean	4	3	6		

Grand mean 4.3

$$SS_{\text{within subjects}} = 1.0 + 0.67 + 4.67 + \ldots = 48.83$$
$$SS_{\text{treatments}} = 5\,[(4\text{-}4.3)^2 + (3\text{-}4.3)^2 + (6\text{-}4.3)^2] = 23.35$$
$$SS_{\text{residual}} = SS_{\text{within subjects}} - SS_{\text{treatments}} = 48.83 - 23.35 = 24.48$$

Source of variation	SS	DF	MS
Within subjects	48.83	10	
Treatments	23.35	2	11.7
Residual	24.48	8	3.1

$$F = \frac{MS_{\text{treatments}}}{MS_{\text{residual}}} = 3.77 \qquad p = 0.20$$

This above table gives an ANOVA table of the data. The table does not permit to conclude, that one of the treatments produces a change. The Bonferroni adjustment of treatments no. 2 and no. 3 of course, does not either ($p = 0.24$ and $p = 0.34$).

In conclusion, with negative correlations between treatment responses statistical methods including paired t-statistics, repeated measures ANOVA, and Bonferroni adjustments for ANOVA lack sensitivity to demonstrate significant treatment effects. The question why this is so, is not difficult to recognize. With t-statistics and a negative correlation between-patient-variation is almost doubled by taking paired differences. With ANOVA things are similar.

$SS_{\text{within subjects}}$ are twice the size of the positive correlation situation while $SS_{\text{treatments}}$ are not different. It follows that the positive correlation situation provides a lot more sensitivity to test than the negative correlation situation does.

1.9.2 Studies Testing Equivalence

In an equivalence trial the conventional significance test has little relevance: failure to detect a difference does not imply equivalence, and a difference, which is detected may not have any clinical relevance and, thus, may not correspond to clinically relevant equivalence. In such trials the range of equivalence is usually predefined as an interval from –D to +D distant from a difference of 0. D is boundary term, and often set equal to a difference of undisputed clinical importance, and hence may be above the minimum of clinical interest by a factor two or three. The bioequivalence study design essentially tests both equivalence and superiority/inferiority. Let us assume that in an equivalence trial of vasodilators for Raynaud's phenomenon 10 patients are treated with vasodilator 1 for one week and for a separate period of one week with vasodilator 2. The data below show the numbers of Raynaud attacks per week.

The underneath table gives correlation levels and their influence on sensitivity of statistical tests.

ρ = -1			ρ = 0			ρ = +1		
vasodilator			vasodilator			vasodilator		
one	two	paired differences	one	two	paired differences	one	two	paired differences
45	10	35	45	40	5	10	10	0
40	15	25	40	35	5	20	15	5
40	15	25	40	35	5	25	15	10
35	20	15	35	30	5	25	20	5
30	25	5	30	25	5	30	25	5
30	25	5	30	10	20	30	25	5
25	30	-5	25	15	10	35	30	5
25	35	-10	25	15	10	40	35	5
20	35	-15	20	20	0	40	35	5
10	40	-30	10	25	-15	40	40	5
means								
30	25	5	30	25	5	30	25	5
SEMs								
3.16	3.16	6.46	3.16	3.16	2.78	3.16	3.16	0.76
t-values								
0.8			1.8			6.3		
95% CIs								
± 14.5			±6.3			± 1.7		

SEM = standard error of the mean;
t means level of t according to t-test for paired differences;
CI means confidence interval calculated according to critical t value of t -distribution for 10-1 pairs = 9 degrees of freedom (critical t = 2.26, 95% CI = 2.26 x SEM);
ρ = correlation coefficient (the Greek letter is often used instead of r if we mean total population instead of our sample).

Although samples have identical means and SEMs (25 ± 3.16 x-axis, 30 ± 3.16 y-axis) their correlation coefficients range from −1 to +1. The null hypothesis of no equivalence is rejected, when the 95% CIs are entirely within the prespecified range of equivalence, in our case defined as between −10 and +10.

In the left trial 95% CIs are between –9.5 and + 19.5, and thus the null hypothesis of no equivalence cannot be rejected. In the middle trial 95% CI are between −1.3 and 11.3, while in the right trial 95% CI are between −3.3 and 6.7. This means, that the last trial has a positive outcome: equivalence is demonstrated, the null hypothesis of no equivalence can be rejected. The negative correlation trial and the zero correlation trial despite a small mean difference between the two treatments, are not sensitive to reject the null-hypothesis, and this is obviously so because of the wide confidence intervals associated with negative and zero correlations.

1.10 Rank Testing

Non-parametric tests are an alternative for ANOVA or t-tests when the data do not have a normal distribution. In that case the former tests are more sensitive than the latter. They are quick and easy, and are based on ranking of data in their order of magnitude. With heavily skewed data this means that we make the distribution of the ranks look a little bit like a normal distribution. We have paired and unpaired non-parametric tests and with the paired test the same problem of loss of sensitivity with negative correlations is encountered as the one we observed with the paired normality tests as discussed in the preceding paragraph. Non-parametric tests are also used to test normal distributions, and provide hardly different results from their parametric counterparts when distributions are approximately normal. Most frequently used tests:

For paired comparisons:

Wilcoxon signed rank test = **paired Wilcoxon** test

For unpaired comparisons:

Mann – Whitney test=**Wilcoxon** rank **sum** test

A paired comparison using Wilcoxon signed rank test is given underneath.

A placebo-controlled clinical trial to test efficacy of sleeping drug is observed.

Patient	Hours of sleep: drug	placebo	difference	rank (ignoring sign)
1	6.1	5.2	0.9	3.5[x]
2	7.0	7.9	-0.9	3.5
3.	8.2	3.9	4.3	10
4.	7.6	4.7	2.9	7
5.	6.5	5.3	1.2	5
6.	8.4	5.4	3.0	8
7.	6.9	4.2	2.7	6
8.	6.7	6.1	0.6	2
9.	7.4	3.8	3.6	9
10.	5.8	6.3	-0.5	1

[x]number 3 and 4 in the rank are tight, so we use 3.5 for both of them.

The Wilcoxon signed rank test uses the signs and the relative magnitudes of the data instead of the actual data. E.g., the above table shows the number of hours sleep in 10 patients tested twice: with sleeping pill and with placebo. We have 3 steps:

1. exclude the differences that are zero, put the remaining differences in ascending order of magnitude and ignore their sign and give them a rank number 1, 2, 3 etc (if differences are equal, average their rank numbers: 3 and 4 become 3.5 and 3.5);
2. add up the positive differences as well as the negative differences;
   + ranknumbers = 3.5+10+7+5+8+6+2+9 = 50.5
   − ranknumbers = 3.5+1 = 4.5
3. The null hypothesis is that there is no difference between + and − ranknumbers. We assess the smaller of the two ranknumbers. The test is significant if the value is smaller than could be expected by chance. We consult the Wilcoxon signed rank table showing us the upper values for 5%, and 1% significance, for the number of differences constituting our rank. In this example we have 10 ranks: 5% and 1% points are respectively 8 and 3. The result is significant at $P < 0.05$, indicating that the sleeping drug is more effective than the placebo.

The table below shows a non/parametric unpaired test called the Mann/Whitney Test. It shows two-samples of patients that are treated with 2 different NSAID agents. Outcome variable is plasma globulin concentration (g/l). Sample one is printed in standard and sample 2 is printed in fat print.

The outcome variable is plasma globulin concentration (g/l). Sample one is printed in standard and sample 2 is printed in fat print.

Globulin concentration(g/l)	ranknumber
26	1
27	**2**
28	**3**
29	4
30	5
31	6
32	7
33	8
34	**9**
35	10
36	11
38	12.5
38	**12.5**
39	**14.5**
39	**14.5**
40	**16**
41	17
42	**18**
45	**19.5**
45	**19.5**

We have 2 steps:

1. The data from both samples are ranked together in ascending order of magnitude. Equal values are averaged.
2. Add up the rank numbers of each of the two samples. In sample-one we have 81.5, in sample-two we have 128.5. We now can consult the Table for Mann-Whitney tests and find with n = 10 and n = 10 (differences in sample sizes are no problem) that the smaller of the two sums of ranks should be smaller than 71 in order to conclude P <0.05. We can, therefore, not reject the null hypothesis of no difference, and have to conclude that the two samples are not significantly different from each other.

1.11 Rank Testing for Three or More Samples

Below an example is given of the data of a Friedman test for paired observations. Paired comparison to test efficacy of 2 dosages of a sleeping drug versus placebo on hours of sleep

Patient	dose 1 (hours)	dose 2	placebo	dose 1 (ranks)	dose 2	placebo
	Hours of sleep					
1	6.1	6.8	5.2	2	3	1
2	7.0	7.0	7.9	1.5	1.5	3
3.	8.2	9.0	3.9	2	3	1
4.	7.6	7.8	4.7	2	3	1
5.	6.5	6.6	5.3	2	3	1
6.	8.4	8.0	5.4	3	2	1
7.	6.9	7.3	4.2	2	3	1
8.	6.7	7.0	6.1	2	3	1
9.	7.4	7.5	3.8	2	3	1
10.	5.8	5.8	6.3	1.5	1.5	3

The Friedman test is used for comparing three or more repeated measures that are not normally distributed, and is an extension of the Wilcoxon signed rank test. An example is given in the table below. The data are ranked for each patient in ascending order of hours of sleep. If the hours are equal, then an average ranknumber is given. Then, for each treatment the squared ranksum is calculated: for dose 1 it equals $(2 + 1.5 + 2 + 2 + 2 + 3 + 2 + 2 + 2 + 1.5)^2 = 400$, for dose 2 it is 676, for placebo it is 196. The following equation is used:

$$\text{chi-square} = \frac{12}{nk\,(k+1)}\left(\text{ranksum}_{dose1}^{2} + \text{ranksum}_{dose2}^{2} + \text{ranksum}_{placebo}^{2}\right) - 3n(k+1)$$

where n = the number of patients and k = the number of treatments.

The chi-square value is calculated to be 7.2. The chi-square statistic will be addressed in Chap. 3. Briefly, it works very similar to the t-statistics. Chi-square values larger than the ones given in the chi-square table in the Appendix indicate that the null-hypothesis of no difference in the data can be rejected. In this example the calculated chi-square value is larger than the rejection chi-square for (3−1) degrees of freedom at $p = 0.05$, and, therefore, we conclude that there is a significant difference between the three treatments at $p < 0.05$. Post-hoc subgroups analyses (using Wilcoxon's tests) are required to find out exactly where the difference is situated, between group 1 and 2, between group 1 and 3, or between group 2 and 3 or between two or more groups. The subject of post-hoc testing is not further discussed here.

Below the data for a Kruskal – Wallis test for unpaired observations is given.

Three-samples of patients are treated with placebo or 2 different NSAIDs (non steroidal anti inflammatory drugs). The outcome variable is the fall in plasma globulin concentration (g/l). Group 1 patients are printed in italics, group 2 in normal standard and group 3 in fat standard print

Globulin concentration(g/l)	ranknumber
-17	***1***
-16	***2***
-5	***3***
-3	***4***
-2	***5***
16	***6***
18	***7***
26	8
27	**9**
28	***10.5***
28	**10.5**
29	12
30	14
30	***14***
30	***14***
31	16
32	17
33	18
34	**19**
35	20
36	21
38	22.5
38	**22.5**
39	**24.5**
39	**24.5**
40	**26**
41	27
42	**28**
45	**29.5**
45	**29.5**

The Kruskal-Wallis test compares multiple groups that are unpaired and not normally distributed, and is an extension of the Mann-Whitney test. Three groups of patients with rheumatoid arthritis are treated with a placebo or one of two different NSAIDs. The fall in plasma globulin (g/l) is used to estimate the effect of treatments. First, we give a ranknumber to every patient dependent on his/her magnitude of fall. If two or three patients have the dame fall, they are given an average ranknumber. Then, we calculate the sum of the ranks for the three groups. For group 1 this amounts to $1 + 2 + 3 + 4 + 5 + 6 + 7 + 10.5 + 14 + 14 = 66.5$, for group 2 to 175.5, group 3 to 488.5. Then we use the equation:

$$\text{chi-square} = \frac{12}{30\,(30-1)}\left(\frac{\text{ranksum}_{group1}^2}{10} + \frac{\text{ranksum}_{group2}^2}{10} + \frac{\text{ranksum}_{group3}^2}{10}\right) - 3(30-1)$$

where the number 30 equals all values, 10 the patient number per group.

The chi-square equals 7744.3. It works very similar to the t-statistics. Briefly, chi-square values larger than the ones given in the underneath chi-square table indicate, that the null-hypothesis of no difference in the data can be rejected (df = degrees of freedom).

	Two-tailed *P*-value			
df	0.10	0.05	0.01	0.001
1	2.706	3.841	6.635	10.827
2	4.605	5.991	9.210	13.815
3	6.251	7.815	11.345	16.266
4	7.779	9.488	13.277	18.466
5	9.236	11.070	15.086	20.515
6	10.645	12.592	16.812	22.457
7	12.017	14.067	18.475	24.321
8	13.362	15.507	20.090	26.124
9	14.684	16.919	21.666	27.877
10	15.987	18.307	23.209	29.588
11	17.275	19.675	24.725	31.264
12	18.549	21.026	26.217	32.909
13	19.812	22.362	27.688	34.527
14	21.064	23.685	29.141	36.124
15	22.307	24.996	30.578	37.698
16	23.542	26.296	32.000	39.252
17	24.769	27.587	33.409	40.791
18	25.989	28.869	34.805	42.312
19	27.204	30.144	36.191	43.819
20	28.412	31.410	37.566	45.314
21	29.615	32.671	38.932	46.796
22	30.813	33.924	40.289	48.268
23	32.007	35.172	41.638	49.728
24	33.196	36.415	42.980	51.179
25	34.382	37.652	44.314	52.619
26	35.563	38.885	45.642	54.051
27	36.741	40.113	46.963	55.475
28	37.916	41.337	48.278	56.892
29	39.087	42.557	49.588	58.301
30	40.256	43.773	50.892	59.702
40	51.805	55.758	63.691	73.403
50	63.167	67.505	76.154	86.660
60	74.397	79.082	88.379	99.608
70	85.527	90.531	100.43	112.32
80	96.578	101.88	112.33	124.84
90	107.57	113.15	124.12	137.21
100	118.50	124.34	135.81	149.45

In this example the calculated chi-square value is much larger than the rejection chi-square for (3−1) degrees of freedom and, therefore, we conclude that there is a significant difference between the three treatments at $p < 0.001$. Post-hoc subgroups analyses (using Man-Whitney tests) are required to find out exactly where the difference is situated, between group 1 and 2, between group 1 and 3, or between group 2 and 3 or between two or more groups.

1.12 Regression Analysis in the Efficacy Analysis of Clinical Trials

Traditionally, regression analyses in clinical were "Not Done", because randomization should be adequate to adjust for confounding. And, if important confounders were to be expected, stratification would be an effective method of adjustment. Nonetheless, the 2013 directives of the EMA (European medicines agency) have addressed the subgroup issue, and have formally noted in its guideline on adjustment, that adjustment in a controlled clinical trial for a few covariates may be considered (European Medicines Agency, April 2013, Doc. EMA/295050/2013).

In the current edition, regressions have been applied. For example, in the Chap. 5 an example is given of a large trial published in a parallel group study in Circulation, which was adjusted for the baseline covariate ldl-cholesterol. Regression analysis is no longer a forbidden methodology in the efficacy analysis of clinical trials.

1.13 Predictors in Clinical Trials

Predictors in clinical trials were, traditionally, treatment modalities, particularly medicines. However, currently, clinical trials are also being performed for the assessment of effects on health and sickness of causal factors other than medicines, for example, effects of interventions like angioplasties, surgeries, renal transplants, special type of care like high altitude treatment in the DAVOS asthma trial (Fieten et al, Trials 2014; 15: 94). Many more factors can be tested in clinical trials, for example,

age factors
psychological factors
social factors
physical factors
economical factors,
and, any factor with a supposedly causal effect on health or sickness.

1.14 Discrete and Discretized Data for Efficacy Analysis

Comparing proportions of responders or proportions of survivors or patients with no events involves binomial rather than normal distributions and requires a completely different approach. It requires a chi-square test, or a more complex technique otherwise closely related to the simple chi-square test, e.g., Mantel Haenszl summary chi-square test, logrank test, Cox proportional hazard test etc. Although in clinical trials, particularly phase III-IV trials, proportions of responders and proportion of survivors is increasingly an efficacy endpoint, in many other trials proportions are used mainly for the purpose of assessing safety endpoints. These methods are summarized widely, particularly in connection with safety analyses, and we will here refer to the recent Springer edition entitled "The Analysis of Safety Data of Drug Trials, an Update, 2019".

Clinical trials are the best way for answering scientific clinical questions. What are the advantages of discrete-data over continuous-data efficacy analysis for answering scientific clinical questions? This question is not easy to answer without having the information about the problem at hand. If the scientific question is a quantitative measure like blood pressure, then a continuous efficacy analysis is the natural choice. However, if the question is of a discrete nature, like, for example, blood pressures higher than 160 mm Hg, then a discrete analysis may provide better data fit. And it seems a matter of course to transform the continuous data for the purpose. Nowadays we have come to recognize that in clinical research the scientific questions are often of a more discrete than continuous nature. For example health scores, quality of life scores, and more health factors are often assessed as discrete levels.

Four more arguments in favor of discretization of continuous variables can be given.

First, clinical data analysis virtually always tries to visualize quantities of raw data. It is, actually, the first step to any numerical analysis.

Second, we live in an era of machine learning, and data mining works with discrete variable spaces.

Third, also traditional efficacy tests, like t-tests, classify trial outcomes into two or more discrete classes.

Fourth, the power of optimal scaling is currently fully recognized, and is another argument in favor of discretization.

Optimal scaling is a method designed to optimize the statistical power of the relationship between the predictor and outcome variables. It makes use of processes like discretization (converting continuous variables into discretized values), and regularization (correcting discretized variables for overfitting, otherwise called overdispersion). This provides better statistics of these data than traditional statistical analysis does.

In clinical trials the research question is often measured with multiple variables. For example, the expressions of a number of genes can be used to predict the efficacy of cytostatic treatment, repeated measurements can be used in randomized longitudinal trials, and multi-item personal scores can be used for the evaluation of antidepressants. Many more examples can be given. Not only t-tests but also regression analyses are often used for analyzing the effect of predictors on outcome variables. The underneath figure gives an example of a continuous predictor variable scored on an outcome scale of 0–10.

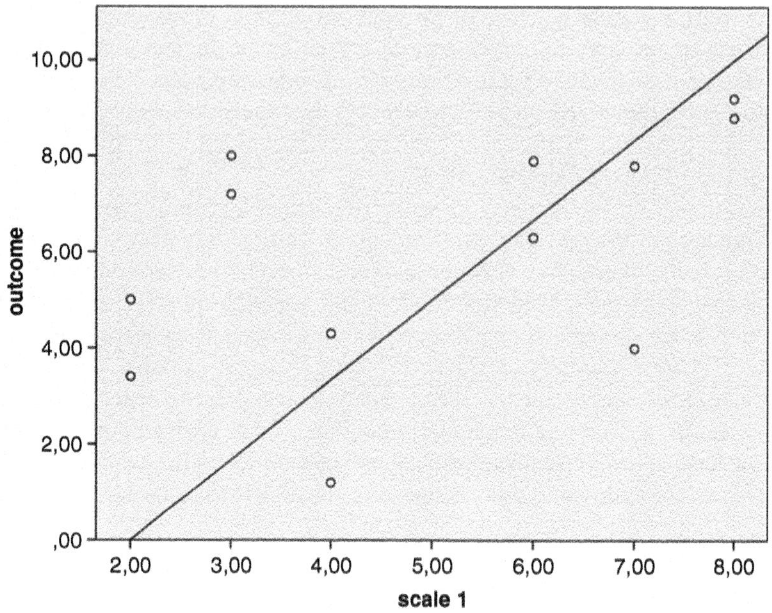

Patients with the predictor values 0, 1, 5, 9 and 10 are missing. Instead of a scale of integers between 0 and 10, other scales are possible, e.g. a scale of two or four scores. Any scale used is, of course, arbitrary and can be replaced with another one.

Scale 1: 0, 1, 2, 3, 4, 5, 6, 7, 8, 9, 10.
Scale 2: 1, 2 (1 = (0–5); 2 = (5–10).
Scale 3: 1, 2, 3, 4 (1 = (0–2.5); 2 = (2.5–5); 3 = (5–7.5); 4 = (7.5–10)

The underneath tables show, that linear regressions of each scale produced different regression coefficients, t-values, and p-values, one result better than the other. With the scales 2 and 3 a gradual improvement of the t-values and p-values is observed. Optimal scaling is a method designed to optimize the statistical power of the relationship between the predictor and outcome variables.

Coefficients[a]

Model		Unstandardized Coefficients		Standardized Coefficients	t	Sig.
		B	Std. Error	Beta		
1	(Constant)	3,351	1,647		2,034	,069
	scale1	,548	,302	,497	1,813	,100

a. Dependent Variable: outcome

Coefficients[a]

Model		Unstandardized Coefficients		Standardized Coefficients	t	Sig.
		B	Std. Error	Beta		
1	(Constant)	2,367	2,032		1,165	,271
	scale2	,497	,257	,521	1,932	,082

a. Dependent Variable: outcome

Coefficients[a]

Model		Unstandardized Coefficients		Standardized Coefficients	t	Sig.
		B	Std. Error	Beta		
1	(Constant)	2,217	1,647		1,346	,208
	scale3	,620	,246	,623	2,520	,030

a. Dependent Variable: outcome

Optimal scaling makes use of processes like discretization (converting continuous variables into discretized values), and regularization (correcting discretized variables for overfitting, otherwise called overdispersion). In order to transform continuous data into a discrete model, the quadratic approximation is convenient: $fx = fa + f^1a\ (x - a)$ where f^1a is the first derivative of the function fa. The quadratic approximation is based on the principle, that the simplest model next to the linear is the quadratic model. Obviously, the magnitude of (any) function can be described by the first derivative of the same function (= slope of the function). This approach is helpful for assessing complex functions like those of standard errors, but also to find the best fit distance (discretization) between some x-value and an x-value close by, called an a-value, which is then used as the best fit scale for the data. In order to further improve the best fit scale for a variable, SPSS provides the possibility to cut a linear variable into two pieces (splines), combining two linear functions for modeling not entirely linear patterns. We should add, that sensitivity of the efficacy analysis can be further maximized by automatic regressions. More information of optimal scaling is in the next chapter.

1.15 Summary of Traditional Methods for Efficacy Analysis Applied in This Edition

Different analytical models were used for traditional efficacy analyses of the clinical trials used as examples in this edition.

Chapter 2: Discretization of continuous predictors

Unpaired t-tests
Simple linear regressions
Multiple linear regressions.
Bonferroni's adjustment

Chapter 3: Confidence intervals

One-way analyses of variance
Kruskal-Wallis tests.

Chapter 4: Confidence intervals

Simple linear regressions.

Chapter 5: Unpaired t-test

Simple linear regressions
Multiple linear regressions.

Chapter 6: Poisson Statistics

Z-tests.

Chapter 7: Linearized model of hyperbola function

Regression model of exponential function.

Chapter 8: Discretization of continuous predictors

Three dimensional bars of effects versus outcome
Crosstabs with chi-square statistics.

Chapter 9: Simple linear regressions

Discretization of continuous predictors
Multiple binary logistic regressions.

Chapter 10: Discretization of continuous predictors

Simple linear regressions.

Chapter 11: Paired t-tests

Confidence intervals
Equivalence testing.

Chapter 12: Discretization of continuous predictors

Crosstabs with chi-square statistics.

Chapter 13: One-way analyses of variance

Multiple linear regressions.

Chapter 14: One-way analyses of variance

3 × 2 Crosstabs with 3 × 2 chi-square statistics
3 Dimensional bars of treatment modalities versus outcomes.

Chapter 15: Discretization of continuous predictors

Crosstabs with chi-square statistics
Multiple binary logistic regressions.

Chapter 16: Discretization of continuous predictors

3 × 2 Crosstabs with 3 × 2 chi-square statistics.

Chapter 17: Discretization of continuous predictors

Crosstabs and chi-square statistics
Multiple binary logistic regressions.

Chapter 18: Simple linear regressions

Multiple linear regressions
Bonferroni's adjustments.

Chapter 19: Simple linear regressions

Multiple linear regressions
Bonferroni's adjustments.

1.16 Summary of Machine Learning Methods for Efficacy Analysis Applied in This Edition

The main objective of the current edition is to assess, for the first time, whether machine learning technologies can be applied for efficacy analysis of controlled clinical trials, and whether it provides advantages. Traditional statistical methods will be tested against important machine learning technologies. The machine learning methods assessed in the current edition are the following.

1. Optimal-Scaling Methods (Chap. 2).
2. Ratio-Statistic Methods (Chap. 3).
3. Complex-Samples Methods (Chap. 4).
4. Bayesian-Network Methods (Chap. 5).

5. Evolutionary-Operation Methods (Chap. 6).
6. Automatic-Newton-Modeling (Chap. 7).
7. High-Risk-Bins Methods (Chap. 8).
8. Balanced-Iterative-Reducing-Hierarchy Methods (Chap. 9).
9. Cluster-Analysis Methods (Chap. 10).
10. Preference-Scoring Methods (Chap. 11)
11. Decision-Tree Methods (Chaps. 12, 13).
12. Automatic-Data-Mining Methods (Chap. 14).
13. Support-Vector-Machine Methods (Chap. 15).
14. Neural-Network Methods (Chap. 16).
15. Ensembled-Accuracy Methods (Chap. 17).
16. Ensembled-Correlation Methods (Chap. 18).
17. Gamma-Distribution Models (Chap. 19).

1.17 Discussion

For the analysis of efficacy data we test null-hypotheses. The t-test is appropriate for two parallel-groups or two paired samples. It is tested, whether one treatment is significantly better than the other, or, with equivalence testing, whether a-priori set boundaries of equivalence are met. Special points with equivalence testing include, the risks of a shift towards a negative study with intention to treat populations and with negative correlations. Analysis of variance (ANOVA) is appropriate for analyzing more than two groups/treatments. For data that do not follow a normal frequency distribution non-parametric tests are available: for paired data the Wilcoxon signed rank or Friedman tests, for unpaired data the Mann-Whitney test or Kruskal-Wallis tests are adequate.

Comparing proportions of responders or proportions of survivors or patients with no events involves binomial rather than normal distributions and requires a completely different approach. It requires a chi-square test, or a more complex technique otherwise closely related to the simple chi-square tests.

Clinical trials are the best way for answering scientific clinical questions. The advantages of discrete-data over continuous-data efficacy analysis for answering scientific clinical questions have been reviewed.

Even better than turning continuous data into discrete ones are scaling machine learning methods which has been reviewed briefly, but will be addressed broadly in the next chapter.

1.18 References

To readers requesting more background, theoretical and mathematical information of computations given, several textbooks complementary to the current production and written by the same authors are available:

Statistics applied to clinical studies 5th edition, 2012,
Machine learning in medicine a complete overview, 2015,
SPSS for starters and 2nd levelers 2nd edition, 2015,
Clinical data analysis on a pocket calculator 2nd edition, 2016,
Understanding clinical data analysis from published research, 2016,
Modern meta-analysis, 2017,
Regression analysis in clinical research, 2018,
Modern Bayesian statistics in clinical research, 2018.
The Analysis of Safety Data of Drug Trials, an Update, 2019.

All of them have been edited by Springer Heidelberg Germany.

Chapter 2
Optimal-Scaling for Efficacy Analysis

Contents

Abstract In a 250 patient self-controlled study of drug efficacy scores, measured as differences from baseline, the effect of highly expressed gene polymorphisms on drug efficacy scores was tested, both traditionally and with the help of machine learning.

Traditional efficacy analysis consisted of

discretization of continuous predictors,
unpaired t-tests,
simple linear regressions,
multiple linear regressions.
Bonferroni's adjustment.

Machine learning efficacy analysis consisted of optimal-scaling methods.

The machine learning methods provided better sensitivity of testing, and were more informative.

Keywords Clinical trials · Traditional efficacy analysis · Machine learning efficacy analysis · Optimal-scaling methods

T. J. Cleophas, A. H. Zwinderman, *Efficacy Analysis in Clinical Trials an Update*,
https://doi.org/10.1007/978-3-030-19918-0_2

2.1 Introduction

Traditional efficacy analyses of clinical trials may consist of unpaired or paired t-tests for testing the significance of difference between the outcome of one treatment versus another, or the significance of difference from baseline in self-controlled studies. Machine learning methods are different, and, rather than means and standard deviations, they test proximities and patterns between data, or, like in the current chapter, they search for optimal scales and shrinkage procedures of your data for better sensitivity of testing. In this chapter a traditional efficacy analysis will be tested against a machine learning methodology called optimal scaling. The traditional efficacy analysis will consist of discretized continuous predictors, unpaired t-tests, simple linear regressions, multiple linear regressions, Bonferroni's adjustments,

2.2 Example

This chapter will use a 250 patient self-controlled study of drug efficacy scores, measured as differences from baseline. The traditional efficacy analysis used simple linear regressions of highly expressed gene levels versus the drug efficacy scores, and step down multiple linear regressions to identify the best fit combination of highly expressed gene levels. The gene expression levels were scored on a scale of 0–10 (VAR = var = variable).

G1	G2	G3	G4	G16	G17	G18	G19	G24	G25	G26	G27	O1	O2	O3	O4
8	8	9	5	7	10	5	6	9	9	6	6	6	7	6	7
9	9	10	9	8	8	7	8	8	9	8	8	8	7	8	7
9	8	8	8	8	9	7	8	9	8	9	9	9	8	8	8
8	9	8	9	6	7	6	4	6	6	5	5	7	7	7	6
10	10	8	10	9	10	10	8	8	9	9	9	8	8	8	7
7	8	8	8	8	7	6	5	7	8	8	7	7	6	6	7
5	5	5	5	5	6	4	5	5	6	6	5	6	5	6	4
9	9	9	9	8	8	8	8	9	8	3	8	8	8	8	8
9	8	9	8	9	8	7	7	7	7	5	8	8	7	6	6
10	10	10	10	10	10	10	10	10	8	8	10	10	10	9	10
2	2	8	5	7	8	8	8	9	3	9	8	7	7	7	6
7	8	8	7	8	6	6	7	8	8	8	7	8	7	8	8
8	9	9	8	10	8	8	7	8	8	9	9	7	7	8	8

Var G1–27 highly expressed genes estimated from their arrays' normalized ratios
Var O1–4 drug efficacy scores (sum of the scores is used as outcome)

Only the data from the first 13 patients are shown. The entire data file entitled "optscaling" can be downloaded from extra.springer.com.

2.3 Traditional Efficacy Analysis

Traditional efficacy analysis consists of t-tests for continuous outcomes and chi-square tests for discrete outcomes. In Sect. 1.12, Chap. 1, the use of regression analyses for efficacy analyses is discussed, and in Sect. 1.13 the use of clinical trials for the assessment of causal health effects of factors other than medicines is discussed. For example, effects of interventions like angioplasties, surgeries, renal transplants etc. Many more factors can be tested in clinical trials, for example,

age factors
psychological factors
social factors
physical factors
economical factors,
and, any factor with a supposedly causal effect on health or sickness.

In the current section SPSS statistical software is used for data analysis. SPSS stands for "statistical package for social sciences", but it is used in multiple disciplines, and will also be used frequently in the current edition. Open the data file in your computer with SPSS installed, and command.

Command:
Analyze....Descriptive Statistics....Descriptives....Variable(s): enter geneone to genetwentyseven....click OK.

The table below is in the output.

Descriptive Statistics

	N	Minimum	Maximum	Mean	Std. Deviation
geneone	250	,00	10,00	7,8040	1,70211
genetwo	250	,00	10,00	7,8040	1,85995
genethree	250	,00	10,00	7,9120	1,78803
genefour	250	3,00	10,00	7,8760	1,52246
genesixteen	250	,00	10,00	7,0520	2,15496
geneseventeen	250	,00	10,00	7,6920	1,80948
geneeighteen	250	,00	10,00	7,1160	2,12806
genenineteen	250	,00	10,00	6,4680	2,22999
genetwentyfour	250	,00	10,00	7,1440	2,60584
genetwentyfive	250	1,00	10,00	7,4040	2,04782
genetwentysix	250	,00	10,00	6,8000	2,66466
genetwentyseven	250	,00	10,00	7,6000	2,27436
Valid N (listwise)	250				

We will use the means as cut-off for discretizing the variable, and transform it into a variable of zeros and ones. Then we will use an unpaired t-test for testing, whether the zeros provide a significantly worse outcome than the ones do.

Command

Transform. . . .Compute Variable. . . .Target Variable: write getwo. . . .Numeric Expression: enter geone. . . .from the blue panel click >. . . .click 7.8. . . .Click OK.

In the data view screen is now a novel variable entitled geone. Subsequently command.

Command

Analyze. . . .Means. . . .Independent-Samples T-Test. . . .Test Variable(s): enter summaryoutcome. . . .Grouping Variable: enter geone. . . .click OK.

The underneath table is in the output.

geneone

Independent Samples Test

		Levene's Test for Equality of Variances		t-test for Equality of Means						
									95% Confidence Interval of the Difference	
		F	Sig.	t	df	Sig. (2-tailed)	Mean Difference	Std. Error Difference	Lower	Upper
summaryoutcome	Equal variances assumed	5,535	,019	-4,805	248	,000	-4,23243	,88081	-5,96726	-2,49761
	Equal variances not assumed			-4,499	136,435	,000	-4,23243	,94072	-6,09271	-2,37215

It shows, that, indeed, the geneone normalized ratios under 7.8 provide a worse drug efficacy score than do those over 7.8, at $p < 0.0001$. The same procedure is followed for all of the predictor genes.

genetwo

Independent Samples Test

		Levene's Test for Equality of Variances		t-test for Equality of Means						
									95% Confidence Interval of the Difference	
		F	Sig.	t	df	Sig. (2-tailed)	Mean Difference	Std. Error Difference	Lower	Upper
summaryoutcome	Equal variances assumed	18,425	,000	-8,380	248	,000	-6,71469	,80127	-8,29286	-5,13652
	Equal variances not assumed			-7,484	129,375	,000	-6,71469	,89724	-8,48985	-4,93952

genethree

Independent Samples Test

		Levene's Test for Equality of Variances		t-test for Equality of Means						
									95% Confidence Interval of the Difference	
		F	Sig.	t	df	Sig. (2-tailed)	Mean Difference	Std. Error Difference	Lower	Upper
summaryoutcome	Equal variances assumed	31,064	,000	-9,753	248	,000	-7,79325	,79910	-9,36715	-6,21936
	Equal variances not assumed			-8,065	98,996	,000	-7,79325	,96627	-9,71054	-5,87597

genefour

Independent Samples Test

		Levene's Test for Equality of Variances		t-test for Equality of Means						
									95% Confidence Interval of the Difference	
		F	Sig.	t	df	Sig. (2-tailed)	Mean Difference	Std. Error Difference	Lower	Upper
summaryoutcome	Equal variances assumed	3,185	,076	-4,963	248	,000	-4,35947	,87831	-6,08936	-2,62957
	Equal variances not assumed			-4,951	159,784	,000	-4,35947	,88043	-6,09825	-2,62068

genesixteen

Independent Samples Test

		Levene's Test for Equality of Variances		t-test for Equality of Means						
									95% Confidence Interval of the Difference	
		F	Sig.	t	df	Sig. (2-tailed)	Mean Difference	Std. Error Difference	Lower	Upper
summaryoutcome	Equal variances assumed	27,613	,000	-9,500	248	,000	-7,03599	,74062	-8,49470	-5,57728
	Equal variances not assumed			-9,616	204,480	,000	-7,03599	,73169	-8,47861	-5,59337

geneseventeen

Independent Samples Test

		Levene's Test for Equality of Variances		t-test for Equality of Means						
									95% Confidence Interval of the Difference	
		F	Sig.	t	df	Sig. (2-tailed)	Mean Difference	Std. Error Difference	Lower	Upper
summaryoutcome	Equal variances assumed	21,641	,000	-10,548	248	,000	-7,91311	,75023	-9,39075	-6,43548
	Equal variances not assumed			-9,606	138,783	,000	-7,91311	,82380	-9,54193	-6,28429

geneeighteen

Independent Samples Test

		Levene's Test for Equality of Variances		t-test for Equality of Means						
									95% Confidence Interval of the Difference	
		F	Sig.	t	df	Sig. (2-tailed)	Mean Difference	Std. Error Difference	Lower	Upper
summaryoutcome	Equal variances assumed	14,429	,000	-7,810	248	,000	-6,05513	,77528	-7,58211	-4,52815
	Equal variances not assumed			-7,718	217,645	,000	-6,05513	,78458	-7,60147	-4,50878

genenineteen

Independent Samples Test

		Levene's Test for Equality of Variances		t-test for Equality of Means						
									95% Confidence Interval of the Difference	
		F	Sig.	t	df	Sig. (2-tailed)	Mean Difference	Std. Error Difference	Lower	Upper
summaryoutcome	Equal variances assumed	28,464	,000	-10,044	248	,000	-7,36258	,73301	-8,80630	-5,91886
	Equal variances not assumed			-9,537	169,677	,000	-7,36258	,77204	-8,88662	-5,83853

genetwentyfour

Independent Samples Test

		Levene's Test for Equality of Variances		t-test for Equality of Means						
									95% Confidence Interval of the Difference	
		F	Sig.	t	df	Sig. (2-tailed)	Mean Difference	Std. Error Difference	Lower	Upper
summaryoutcome	Equal variances assumed	24,582	,000	-11,634	248	,000	-8,79522	,75600	-10,28423	-7,30621
	Equal variances not assumed			-9,716	100,546	,000	-8,79522	,90524	-10,59107	-6,99937

genetwentyfive

Independent Samples Test

		Levene's Test for Equality of Variances		t-test for Equality of Means						
									95% Confidence Interval of the Difference	
		F	Sig.	t	df	Sig. (2-tailed)	Mean Difference	Std. Error Difference	Lower	Upper
summaryoutcome	Equal variances assumed	3,906	,049	-5,386	248	,000	-4,45272	,82680	-6,08115	-2,82428
	Equal variances not assumed			-5,269	207,916	,000	-4,45272	,84512	-6,11882	-2,78661

genetwentysix

Independent Samples Test

		Levene's Test for Equality of Variances		t-test for Equality of Means						
									95% Confidence Interval of the Difference	
		F	Sig.	t	df	Sig. (2-tailed)	Mean Difference	Std. Error Difference	Lower	Upper
summaryoutcome	Equal variances assumed	23,623	,000	-10,499	248	,000	-7,95079	,75726	-9,44227	-6,45932
	Equal variances not assumed			-9,209	122,731	,000	-7,95079	,86341	-9,65991	-6,24168

genetwentyseven

Independent Samples Test

		Levene's Test for Equality of Variances		t-test for Equality of Means						
									95% Confidence Interval of the Difference	
		F	Sig.	t	df	Sig. (2-tailed)	Mean Difference	Std. Error Difference	Lower	Upper
summaryoutcome	Equal variances assumed	,116	,733	-4,778	248	,000	-4,09006	,85597	-5,77597	-2,40416
	Equal variances not assumed			-4,940	213,399	,000	-4,09006	,82797	-5,72211	-2,45801

Obviously, all of the unpaired t-tests were very significant. The univariate analyses indicate, that all of the genes are very good predictors of drug efficacy. However interaction between the genes is not taken into account in these simple analyses, and this may very well have overestimated the above results. In order to adjust confounding and interaction, regression analysis is appropriate, and it is approved by the EMA, even for the primary data analysis of clinical trials (European Medicines Agency, April 2013, Doc. EMA/295050/2013). Therefore, a regression analysis was, subsequently, performed. First construct a novel variable entitled summaryoutcome.

Command
click Transform. . . .click ComputeVariable. . . .Target Variable: write summaryoutcome. . . .Numeric Expression: outcomeone. . . .in blue field click +. . . . outcometwo. . . .in blue field click +. . . .outcomethree. . . .in blue field click+. . . . outcomefour. . . .click OK.

In the data view screen a novel variable entitled summaryoutcome is observed.

Command
Analyze. . . .Regression. . . .Linear. . . .Dependent: enter summaryoutcome. . . . Independent: enter the 12 highly expressed genes one by one. . . .click OK.

In the output sheets the underneath tables are given.

Coefficients[a]

Model		Unstandardized Coefficients		Standardized Coefficients	t	Sig.
		B	Std. Error	Beta		
1	(Constant)	15,083	1,870		8,064	,000
	geneone	1,570	,234	,392	6,702	,000

a. Dependent Variable: summaryoutcome

Coefficients[a]

Model		Unstandardized Coefficients		Standardized Coefficients	t	Sig.
		B	Std. Error	Beta		
1	(Constant)	10,252	1,499		6,838	,000
	genetwo	2,189	,187	,597	11,709	,000

a. Dependent Variable: summaryoutcome

Coefficients[a]

Model		Unstandardized Coefficients		Standardized Coefficients	t	Sig.
		B	Std. Error	Beta		
1	(Constant)	7,938	1,506		5,271	,000
	genethree	2,451	,186	,642	13,201	,000

a. Dependent Variable: summaryoutcome

Coefficients[a]

Model		Unstandardized Coefficients		Standardized Coefficients	t	Sig.
		B	Std. Error	Beta		
1	(Constant)	15,319	2,146		7,138	,000
	genefour	1,525	,268	,340	5,700	,000

a. Dependent Variable: summaryoutcome

Coefficients[a]

Model		Unstandardized Coefficients		Standardized Coefficients	t	Sig.
		B	Std. Error	Beta		
1	(Constant)	10,733	,991		10,829	,000
	genesixteen	2,354	,134	,743	17,507	,000

a. Dependent Variable: summaryoutcome

Coefficients[a]

Model		Unstandardized Coefficients		Standardized Coefficients	t	Sig.
		B	Std. Error	Beta		
1	(Constant)	7,882	1,403		5,617	,000
	geneseventeen	2,529	,178	,671	14,239	,000

a. Dependent Variable: summaryoutcome

Coefficients[a]

Model		Unstandardized Coefficients		Standardized Coefficients	t	Sig.
		B	Std. Error	Beta		
1	(Constant)	15,194	1,280		11,870	,000
	geneeighteen	1,706	,172	,532	9,895	,000

a. Dependent Variable: summaryoutcome

Coefficients[a]

Model		Unstandardized Coefficients		Standardized Coefficients	t	Sig.
		B	Std. Error	Beta		
1	(Constant)	13,708	,964		14,224	,000
	genenineteen	2,106	,141	,688	14,950	,000

a. Dependent Variable: summaryoutcome

Coefficients[a]

Model		Unstandardized Coefficients		Standardized Coefficients	t	Sig.
		B	Std. Error	Beta		
1	(Constant)	14,999	,950		15,785	,000
	genetwentyfour	1,726	,125	,659	13,813	,000

a. Dependent Variable: summaryoutcome

Coefficients[a]

Model		Unstandardized Coefficients		Standardized Coefficients	t	Sig.
		B	Std. Error	Beta		
1	(Constant)	17,522	1,491		11,753	,000
	genetwentyfive	1,325	,194	,398	6,826	,000

a. Dependent Variable: summaryoutcome

Coefficients[a]

Model		Unstandardized Coefficients		Standardized Coefficients	t	Sig.
		B	Std. Error	Beta		
1	(Constant)	15,964	,899		17,756	,000
	genetwentysix	1,672	,123	,653	13,576	,000

a. Dependent Variable: summaryoutcome

Coefficients[a]

Model		Unstandardized Coefficients		Standardized Coefficients	t	Sig.
		B	Std. Error	Beta		
1	(Constant)	19,495	1,419		13,741	,000
	genetwentyseven	1,031	,179	,344	5,765	,000

a. Dependent Variable: summaryoutcome

Obviously, all of the above univariate linear regressions were statistically very significant with t-values from 5.8 to 17.0. However, dependencies between the predicting gene levels were not accounted in the analyses so far. Therefore, a step down multiple linear regression was in the protocol, and was, subsequently, performed.

Command

Analyze. . . .Regression. . . .Linear. . . .Dependent: enter the summary scores of the 4 outcome variables (use Transform and Compute Variable command). . . . Independent: enter the 12 highly expressed genes simultaneously . . . .click OK.

In the output sheets the underneath table was given.

Coefficients[a]

Model		Unstandardized Coefficients B	Unstandardized Coefficients Std. Error	Standardized Coefficients Beta	t	Sig.
1	(Constant)	3,293	1,475		2,232	,027
	geneone	-,122	,189	-,030	-,646	,519
	genetwo	,287	,225	,078	1,276	,203
	genethree	,370	,228	,097	1,625	,105
	genefour	,063	,196	,014	,321	,748
	genesixteen	,764	,172	,241	4,450	,000
	geneseventeen	,835	,198	,221	4,220	,000
	geneeighteen	,088	,151	,027	,580	,563
	genenineteen	,576	,154	,188	3,751	,000
	genetwentyfour	,403	,146	,154	2,760	,006
	genetwentyfive	,028	,141	,008	,198	,843
	genetwentysix	,320	,142	,125	2,250	,025
	genetwentyseven	-,275	,133	-,092	-2,067	,040

a. Dependent Variable: summaryoutcome

The number of statistically significant p-values (indicated here with Sig.), < 0.10 was in 6 out of 12. In order to improve this result, the insignificant predictors were subsequently deleted from the model. And the same commands were given once more. This left us with the model in the underneath table.

Coefficients[a]

Model		Unstandardized Coefficients B	Unstandardized Coefficients Std. Error	Standardized Coefficients Beta	t	Sig.
1	(Constant)	5,438	1,118		4,864	,000
	genesixteen	,883	,167	,279	5,282	,000
	geneseventeen	,933	,180	,248	5,186	,000
	genenineteen	,721	,147	,236	4,913	,000
	genetwentyfour	,452	,146	,173	3,099	,002
	genetwentysix	,369	,139	,144	2,655	,008
	genetwentyseven	-,252	,127	-,084	-1,990	,048

a. Dependent Variable: summaryoutcome

In the model above 6 insignificant predictors were deleted, and 6 significant ones were maintained. Many very independent determinants were thus maintained in the final model, although interaction tests were not yet included in the model.

With Bonferroni correction for multiple testing the rejection type I error (alpha) of 0.05 should be reduced to with number of statistical tests of k = 6

$$\begin{aligned}\text{alpha corrected} &= \text{alpha} \times [2/k(k-1)] \\ &= 0.05 \times \big(2/(6 \times 5) \\ &= 0.00333\end{aligned}$$

This would mean, that the genetwentysix and -twentyseven were not statistically significant anymore.

2.4 Optimal Scaling for Efficacy Analysis

In order to try and improve this result, a scaling machine learning method was applied. Continuous predictor variables were converted into best fit discretized ones. SPSS was used again. The underneath commands were given.

Command
Analyze....Regression....Optimal Scaling....Dependent Variable: Var 28 (Define Scale: mark spline ordinal 2.2)....Independent Variables: Var 1, 2, 3, 4, 16, 17, 18, 19, 24, 25, 26, 27 (all of them Define Scale: mark spline ordinal 2.2).... Discretize: Method Grouping)....OK.

The table below was in the output sheets.

Coefficients

	Standardized Coefficients		df	F	Sig.
	Beta	Bootstrap (1000) Estimate of Std. Error			
geneone	-,109	,110	2	,988	,374
genetwo	,193	,107	3	3,250	,023
genethree	-,092	,119	2	,591	,555
genefour	,113	,074	3	2,318	,077
genesixteen	,263	,087	4	9,065	,000
geneseventeen	,301	,114	2	6,935	,001
geneeighteen	,113	,136	1	,687	,408
genenineteen	,145	,067	1	4,727	,031
genetwentyfour	,220	,097	2	5,166	,007
genetwentyfive	-,039	,094	1	,170	,681
genetwentysix	,058	,107	2	,293	,746
genetwentyseven	-,127	,104	2	1,490	,228

Dependent Variable: summaryoutcome

There is no intercept anymore, and the t-tests have been replaced with F-tests. The optimally scaled model can be improved with some kind of regularization. Regularization can be defined as a method for correcting discretized variables for overfitting, otherwise called overdispersion.

The number of p-values < 0.10 is in 6 out of 12. In order to fully benefit from optimal scaling a number of regularization procedures for the purpose of correcting overdispersion (more spread in the data than compatible with Gaussian data) are possible. Ridge regression minimizes the b-values such that $b_{ridge} = b/(1+\text{shrinking factor})$. With shrinking factor $= 0$, $b_{ridge} = b$, with ∞, $b_{ridge} = 0$. First, optimal scaling with ridge regression was performed.

Command

Analyze....Regression....Optimal Scaling....Dependent Variable: Var 28 (Define Scale: mark spline ordinal 2.2)....Independent Variables: Var 1, 2, 3, 4, 16, 17, 18, 19, 24, 25, 26, 27 (all of them Define Scale: mark spline ordinal 2.2).... Discretize: Method Grouping, Number categories 7)....click Regularization.... mark Ridge....click OK.

Coefficients

	Standardized Coefficients		df	F	Sig.
	Beta	Bootstrap (1000) Estimate of Std. Error			
geneone	,032	,033	2	,946	,390
genetwo	,068	,021	3	10,842	,000
genethree	,051	,030	1	2,963	,087
genefour	,064	,020	3	10,098	,000
genesixteen	,139	,024	4	34,114	,000
geneseventeen	,142	,025	2	31,468	,000
geneeighteen	,108	,040	2	7,236	,001
genenineteen	,109	,020	2	30,181	,000
genetwentyfour	,109	,021	2	27,855	,000
genetwentyfive	,041	,038	3	1,178	,319
genetwentysix	,098	,023	2	17,515	,000
genetwentyseven	-,017	,047	1	,132	,716

Dependent Variable: 20-23

The sensitivity of this model is better than the above two methods with 7 p-values < 0.0001, and 9 p-values < 0.10, while the traditional and unregularized Optimal Scaling only produced 6 and 6 p-values < 0.10. Also the lasso regularization model is possible (Var = variable). It shrinks the small b values to 0. Second, optimal scaling with lasso regression was performed.

Command

Analyze....Regression....Optimal Scaling....Dependent Variable: Var 28 (Define Scale: mark spline ordinal 2.2)....Independent Variables: Var 1, 2, 3, 4, 16, 17, 18, 19, 24, 25, 26, 27 (all of them Define Scale: mark spline ordinal 2.2).... Discretize: Method Grouping, Number categories 7)....click Regularization.... mark Lasso....click OK.

Coefficients

	Standardized Coefficients				
	Beta	Bootstrap (1000) Estimate of Std. Error	df	F	Sig.
geneone	,000	,020	0	,000	.
genetwo	,054	,046	3	1,390	,247
genethree	,000	,026	0	,000	.
genefour	,011	,036	3	,099	,960
genesixteen	,182	,084	4	4,684	,001
geneseventeen	,219	,095	3	5,334	,001
geneeighteen	,086	,079	2	1,159	,316
genenineteen	,105	,063	2	2,803	,063
genetwentyfour	,124	,078	2	2,532	,082
genetwentyfive	,000	,023	0	,000	.
genetwentysix	,048	,060	2	,647	,525
genetwentyseven	,000	,022	0	,000	.

Dependent Variable: 20-23

The b-values of the genes 1, 3, 25 and 27 are now shrunk to zero, and eliminated from the analysis. Lasso is particularly suitable if you are looking for a limited number of predictors and improves prediction accuracy by leaving out weak predictors. Finally, the elastic net method is applied. Like lasso it shrinks the small b-values to 0, but it performs better with many predictor variables. Third, optimal scaling with elastic net regression was performed.

Command

Analyze. . . .Regression. . . .Optimal Scaling. . . .Dependent Variable: Var 28 (Define Scale: mark spline ordinal 2.2). . . .Independent Variables: Var 1, 2, 3, 4, 16, 17, 18, 19, 24, 25, 26, 27 (all of them Define Scale: mark spline ordinal 2.2). . . . Discretize: Method Grouping, Number categories 7). . . .click Regularization. . . . mark Elastic Net. . . .click OK.

Coefficients

	Standardized Coefficients				
	Beta	Bootstrap (1000) Estimate of Std. Error	df	F	Sig.
geneone	,000	,016	0	,000	.
genetwo	,029	,039	3	,553	,647
genethree	,000	,032	3	,000	1,000
genefour	,000	,015	0	,000	.
genesixteen	,167	,048	4	12,265	,000
geneseventeen	,174	,051	3	11,429	,000
geneeighteen	,105	,055	2	3,598	,029
genenineteen	,089	,048	3	3,420	,018
genetwentyfour	,113	,053	2	4,630	,011
genetwentyfive	,000	,012	0	,000	.
genetwentysix	,062	,046	2	1,786	,170
genetwentyseven	,000	,018	0	,000	.

Dependent Variable: 20-23

The results are pretty much the same, as it is with lasso. Elastic net does not provide additional benefit in this example, but it works better than lasso if the number of predictors is larger than the number of observations.

Optimal scaling of linear regression data, thus, provided little benefit due to overdispersion. However, regularized optimal scaling using ridge regression provided excellent results. Lasso optimal scaling was also suitable, particularly if you were looking for a limited number of strong predictors. Elastic net optimal scaling worked better than lasso, particularly, if the number of predictors was large.

2.5 Discussion

Traditional efficacy analyses of clinical trials may consist of unpaired or paired t-tests for testing the significance of difference between the outcome of one treatment versus another, or the significance of difference from baseline in self-controlled studies. Machine learning methods are different, and, rather than means and standard deviations, they assess proximities and patterns between data, or, like in the current chapter, they search for optimal scales and shrinkage procedures of your data for better sensitivity of testing.

Optimal scaling of linear regression data provided, however, little benefit due to overdispersion. In contrast, regularized optimal scaling using ridge regression provided excellent results. Lasso optimal scaling was also suitable, particularly if you were looking for a limited number of strong predictors. Elastic net optimal scaling worked better than lasso, if the number of predictors was large.

In this chapter traditional efficacy analysis consistent of

discretized continuous predictors,
unpaired t-tests,
simple linear regressions,
multiple linear regressions,
Bonferroni's adjustments,

were tested against a machine learning methodology called optimal scaling. Optimal scaling, particularly, if regularized with ridge regression, provided excellent results of efficacy analysis, and better so than traditional efficacy analysis.

The machine learning efficacy analyses included optimal scaling methodologies. The machine learning analyses provided better sensitivity of testing, and were more informative.

2.6 References

More information of optimal scaling with or without regularization is available in Machine learning in medicine part one, Chapters 3 and 4, entitled "Optimal scaling: discretization", and "Optimal scaling: regularization including ridge, lasso, and elastic net regression", pp 25–37, and pp 39–53, Springer Heidelberg Germany, 2013, from the same authors.

To readers requesting more background, theoretical and mathematical information of computations given, several textbooks complementary to the current production and also written by the same authors are available:

Statistics applied to clinical studies 5th edition, 2012,
Machine learning in medicine a complete overview, 2015,
SPSS for starters and 2nd levelers 2nd edition, 2015,
Clinical data analysis on a pocket calculator 2nd edition, 2016,
Understanding clinical data analysis from published research, 2016,
Modern meta-analysis, 2017,
Regression analysis in clinical research, 2018,
Modern Bayesian statistics in clinical research, 2018.
The analysis of safety data of drug trials an update, 2019.

All of them have been edited by Springer Heidelberg Germany.

Chapter 3
Ratio-Statistic for Efficacy Analysis

Contents

Abstract In a 50 patient parallel-group trial, the effects of treatment modalities on baseline minus treatment cholesterol level was tested, both traditionally and with the help of machine learning.

Traditional efficacy analysis was consisted of

confidence intervals,
one-way analyses of variance,
Kruskal-Wallis tests.

Machine learning efficacy analysis consisted of ratio-statistic methods.

The machine learning methods provided better sensitivity of testing, and were more informative.

Keywords Clinical trials · Traditional efficacy analysis · Machine learning efficacy analysis · Ratio-statistic methods

3.1 Introduction

Typical efficacy endpoints have their associated statistical techniques. Values of continuous measurements (e.g., blood pressures) require the following statistical techniques:

(a) if measurements are normally distributed: t-tests and associated confidence intervals to compare two mean values; analysis of variance (ANOVA) to compare three or more,

T. J. Cleophas, A. H. Zwinderman, *Efficacy Analysis in Clinical Trials an Update*,
https://doi.org/10.1007/978-3-030-19918-0_3

(b) if measurements have a non-normal distribution: Wilcoxon or Mann-Whitney tests with confidence intervals for medians, Friedman or Kruskal-Wallis for three or more groups.

Treatment efficacies are often assessed as differences from baseline. However, better treatment efficacies may be observed in patients with high baseline-values than in those with low ones. This was, e.g., the case in the Progress study, a parallel-group study of pravastatin versus placebo (Chap. 17, Statistics Applied to Clinical Studies Fifth Edition, Springer Heidelberg Germany, 2012, from the same authors). Machine learning methods may provide better sensitivity of testing than traditional methods may. This chapter tests the performance of traditional efficacy analysis against a machine learning method called ratio-statistic. The traditional efficacy analysis consists of one way analyses of variance and Kruskal-Wallis tests.

3.2 Data Example

The differences of treatment efficacy and baseline may be the best fit test statistic, if the treatment efficacies are independent of baseline. However, if not, then ratios of the two may fit the data better.

In 50 patients a five-group parallel-group trial was performed with five different cholesterol-lowering compounds. The first 12 patients of the data file is underneath. The entire data file is entitled "ratiostatistic" and is in extra.springer.com.

Variable 1 Baseline	Variable 2 Treatment	Variable 3 Treatment	Variable 4 "baseline minus treatment"
cholesterol (mmol/l)	cholesterol (mmol/l)	group no.	cholesterol level (mmol/l)
6.10	5.20	1.00	.90
7.00	7.90	1.00	-.90
8.20	3.90	1.00	4.30
7.60	4.70	1.00	2.90
6.50	5.30	1.00	1.20
8.40	5.40	1.00	3.00
6.90	4.20	1.00	2.70
6.70	6.10	1.00	.60
7.40	3.80	1.00	3.60
5.80	6.30	1.00	-.50
6.20	4.30	2.00	1.90
7.10	6.80	2.00	.30

Start by opening the above data file in your computer with SPSS statistical software installed.

Command

Graphs....Legacy Dialogs.....Error Bar....mark Summaries of groups of cases.... click Define....Variable: enter "baseline minus treatment"....Category Axis: enter Treatment group....Confidence interval for mean: Level enter 95%....click OK.

The underneath graph shows, that all of the treatments were excellent, and significantly lowered cholesterol levels, as shown by the 95% confidence intervals. The differences are such, that a significant difference from zero can be read from the graph, and t-tests are not even needed.

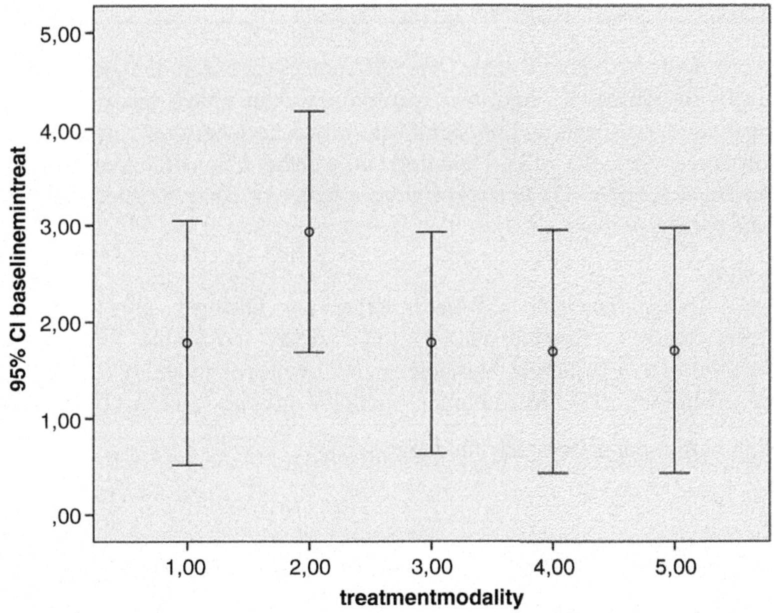

3.3 Traditional Efficacy Analysis

In order to assess, whether any of the treatments significantly outperformed the others, a one-way analysis of variance (ANOVA), with treatment modality as predictor and "baseline minus treatment" as outcome, was performed. Again SPSS statistical software was applied.

Command
Analyze....Compare means....One-Way ANOVA....Dependent List: enter "base-line mintreat"....Factor: enter treatment modality....click OK.

In the output sheets the underneath table is displayed.

ANOVA

baselinemintreat

	Sum of Squares	df	Mean Square	F	Sig.
Between Groups	10,603	4	2,651	,886	,480
Within Groups	134,681	45	2,993		
Total	145,284	49			

According to the above table, the differences between the treatments were statistically insignificant. And, so, according to the above analysis, all of the treatment were excellent, and no significant differences between any of the groups were observed. Next, we will try and find out, whether a non-Gaussian alternative to the above unpaired ANOVA test provides a better p-value. Kruskal-Wallis test is adequate for the purpose.

Command
Analyze....Nonparametric Tests....Legacy Dialogs....K Independent Samples....mark Kruskal-Wallis H....Test Variable List: enter baselinemintreat....Grouping Variable: enter treatment modality....click Define Range....Minimum:1....Maximum:5....click Continue....click OK.

In the output the underneath table are given.

Ranks

	treatmentmodality	N	Mean Rank
baselinemintreat	1,00	10	24,70
	2,00	9	33,72
	3,00	11	24,00
	4,00	10	23,00
	5,00	10	23,05
	Total	50	

Test Statistics[a,b]

	baselinemintreat
Chi-Square	3,591
df	4
Asymp. Sig.	,464

a. Kruskal Wallis Test
b. Grouping Variable: treatmentmodality

The p-value is smaller but still far from significant. Next, we will assess, whether with Ratio-Statistic Methods additional and better sensitive results can be obtained.

3.4 Ratio-Statistic for Efficacy Analysis

Ratio-Statistic Methods are available in SPSS statistical software in the module Descriptive Statistics. The underneath commands are required.

Command

Analyze....Descriptive Statistics....Ratio....Numerator: enter "treatment".... Denominator: enter "baseline"....Group Variable: enter "treatment modality (treatment group)"....click Statistics....mark Median....mark COD (coefficient of dispersion)....Concentration Index: Low Proportion: type 0.8....High Proportion: type 1.2....click Add....Percent of Median: enter 20....click Add....click Continue....click OK.

The underneath table is now shown in the output sheets.

Ratio Statistics for treatment / baseline

			Coefficient of Concentration	
Group	Median	Coefficient of Dispersion	Percent between 0.8 and 1.2 inclusive	Within 20% of Median inclusive
1.00	.729	.265	50.0%	50.0%
2.00	.597	.264	22.2%	44.4%
3.00	.663	.269	36.4%	54.5%
4.00	.741	.263	50.0%	50.0%
5.00	.733	.267	50.0%	50.0%
Overall	.657	.282	42.0%	38.0%

A problem with ratios is, that they, usually, suffer from overdispersion, and, therefore, the spread in the data must be assessed differently from that of normal distributions. First, medians are applied, which is not the mean value, but the values in the middle of all values. Assessment of spread is, then, estimated with

II. the coefficient of dispersion
III. the percentual coefficient of concentration (all ratios within 20% of the median are included)
IIII. the interval coefficient of concentration (all ratios between the ratio 0.8 $*$ median, and 1.2 $*$ median are included ($*$ = symbol of multiplication).

If the distribution of the ratios are very skewed, then the coefficients II and III are not the same. The above table, thus, shows the following.

Obviously, the treatment 2 performs best with 60% reduction of cholesterol after treatment.

The treatment 5 performs worst with only 74% reduction of cholesterol after treatment.

The coefficient I is a general measure of variability of the ratios, and the coefficient III shows the same, but is easier to interpret:

around 50% Of the individual ratios are within 20% distance from the median ratio.

The coefficient II gives the percentage of individual ratios:

between the interval of 0.8 $*$ and 1.2 $*$ the median ratio.

Particularly, the groups 2 and 3 have small coefficients, indicating little concentration of the individual ratios here. The group 2 may produce the best median ratio, but is also the least concentrated, and is, thus, more uncertain than, for example, the groups 1, 4, 5.

It would make sense, from these observations, to conclude, that treatment- group 1, with more certainty, is a better treatment choice than treatment group 2 is.

3.5 Discussion

The traditional ANOVAs and Kruskal-Wallis tests for efficacy analysis of the parallel-group trial in this chapter did not produce any difference between the efficacies of five treatment modalities. The ratio-statistic Method did not produce any p-value either. Yet, we were able to conclude, that one treatment was a better and more certain choice than the others.

Treatment efficacies are often assessed as differences from baseline. However, better treatment efficacies may be observed in patients with high baseline-values than in those with low ones. The differences of treatment efficacy and baseline may be the best fit test statistic, if the treatment efficacies are independent of baseline. However, if not, then ratios of the two may better fit the data, and allow for relevant additional support against the null-hypothesis of no differences.

In this chapter the traditional efficacy analysis consisted of confidence intervals, one-way analyses of variance, and Kruskal-Wallis tests, and the machine learning analyses included ratio statistic methods. The machine learning analyses provided better sensitivity of testing, and were more informative.

3.6 References

To readers requesting more background, theoretical and mathematical information of computations given, several textbooks complementary to the current production and written by the same authors are available:

Statistics applied to clinical studies 5th edition, 2012,
Machine learning in medicine a complete overview, 2015,
SPSS for starters and 2nd levelers 2nd edition, 2015,
Clinical data analysis on a pocket calculator 2nd edition, 2016,
Understanding clinical data analysis from published research, 2016,
Modern meta-analysis, 2017,
Regression analysis in clinical research, 2018,
Modern Bayesian statistics in clinical research, 2018.
The Analysis of Safety Data of Drug Trials, an Update, 2019.

All of them have been edited by Springer Heidelberg Germany.

Chapter 4
Complex-Samples for Efficacy Analysis

Contents

Abstract In a 1000 person random sample, the effects of time and territorial divisions on health scores were tested, both traditionally, and with the help of machine learning.

Traditional efficacy analysis consisted of

confidence intervals,
simple linear regressions.

Machine learning efficacy analysis consisted of complex-samples methods.

The machine learning methods provided better sensitivity of testing, and were more informative.

Keywords Clinical trials · Traditional efficacy analysis · Machine learning efficacy analysis · Complex-samples methods

4.1 Introduction

A real data example of the problems with the analysis of big data is in the 2000 National Institute of Health study of health parameters of the USA citizens including smoking habits, vitamin and mineral supplies, multivitamin consumption, body weight, daily exercise information, and herbal supplies. The study included about 0.3 billion of inhabitants, and census information was used to obtain most of the values of different states, city districts, and even townships and neighborhoods.

T. J. Cleophas, A. H. Zwinderman, *Efficacy Analysis in Clinical Trials an Update*,
https://doi.org/10.1007/978-3-030-19918-0_4

However, little was known about the health parameters. It was decided to randomly sample 30,000 inhabitants throughout the country as a representative sample of the entire population, and these data could be used for comparisons between states, cities and other subgroups. However, it was recognized that different parts of the country would have different probabilities of being included in the sample. First, the states were not equally sized, and, thus, larger states had a larger chance of including individuals. Second, the sampled individuals were taken from different cities and city districts, and these were again different in probability of being included. For these differences probability corrections had to be performed and a correction factor, otherwise called weighting factor, had to be added to each individual in the sample prior to data analysis. Such a complex analysis is hard to accomplish without complex sampling procedures.

Health scores, including measures of physical, mental and social health are increasingly considered important to estimate public health. If in one territorial division 40% has a low health score, and in another equally large territorial divisions 60%, then on average 50% has a low health score. If the first territorial division is larger than the second, e.g. 1.5 times larger (with similar population density), then we have 1.5 times larger chance that an individual from the 40% low scores is sampled. This would mean that, instead of an average of 50% low health scores for the two territorial divisions,

$$(1/2 \times 40 + 1/2 \times 60)/2 = 50\%,$$

the following average will be measured:

$$(3/5 \times 40 + 2/5 \times 60)/2 = 48\%.$$

This result is 2 % smaller, and this is due to the difference in size of the two territorial divisions. Complex sample methodology adjusts these kinds of effects by adding appropriate weights to the individual data. However, with experimental data, uncertainty should be taken into account, and this is also true for the weights to be added as a multiplication factor to the individuals' data. This complicates statistical analyses. Different mathematical methods are available for adjusting the biased estimations. The replication method randomly selects a set of subsamples from the sampled data and overall estimates are computed from them. The Jack-knife method works similarly and calculates means and variances by repeatedly deleting one measured value. Both are Monte Carlo methods and can be applied without the need to take account of theoretical data distribution patterns. They are, respectively, used in SPSS with proportional and numeric data. Taylor series makes use of the algebraic phenomenon that any function f(x) can be expressed as the sum of another function f(a) and its derivative times $(x–a)^2$. It enables to account and compute the variances of ratio data and weighted ratios. We should add that computations are further complicated by the repeated nature of many observations in population studies, requiring paired analyses, and accounting, not only the variances but also the co-variances in the data.

In this chapter efficacy analyses of the effects of territorial divisions and of time on population health scores were assessed. Traditional efficacy analysis will be tested against a machine learning methodology entitled complex-samples methodology. The traditional efficacy analysis consists of confidence intervals, and simple linear regressions.

4.2 Data Example

Population scores like financial, physical, mental, social and many other types of scores are the subject of study not only by governments and public authorities, but also by major commercial institutions like pharmaceutical companies, health organizations and other research groups. Objectives include prediction purposes, the allocation of resources and others. The research of entire populations is laborious and obtaining information from representative samples instead of an entire population is more time- and cost-efficient. However, this method is generally biased, because each individual selected is given the same probability of being selected. Complex sample technology is particularly suitable for that purpose, because it produces largely unbiased population estimates. This, however, requires special sampling techniques taking into account the different probabilities of individuals being included in a population-based survey. It is a computationally intensive method that calculates weighting factors for the individuals included. The current paper uses a hypothesized example of a 9678 member population health scores, and is supposed to assess the improvements in the past few years. The results of complex sample analyses and those of traditional analyses are compared. SPSS statistical software is applied for all of the analyses. For the benefit of students step be step analyses will be given.

Prior health scores of a 9678 member population recorded some 5–10 years ago were supposed to be available, as well as topographical information. We wish to obtain information of the current versus the prior health scores, using complex samples methodology. For that purpose the information of the entire data plus additional information on the current health scores from a random sample of 1000 from this population were used. The region consisted of four territorial divisions, 88 townships and 613 neighborhoods. First, a sampling plan was designed.

Then, a random sample of 1000 was taken and additional information was obtained, and included in the data file. The data file plus the sampling plan were, then, used for various complex-samples analyses. Also the results of traditional and the complex-samples analyses were compared. The SPSS modules complex samples (cs) descriptives, cs general linear model, and cs ratios were applied, as well as the appropriate modules for the traditional analyses.

Population data summary

Population	9,678 cases
Territorial divisions	4
Townships	88
Neighborhoods	613
Stage 1 sampling plan	the counties are the strata, the townships are the clusters 4 clusters / stratum
Stage 2 sampling plan	the neighborhoods are the strata the cases are the clusters (clusters of one) a proportion of 0.2 of the cases clustered / stratum

A sampling plan of the above population data is designed using SPSS. Open in extras.springer.com the database entitled "healthscores_cs". The territorial divisions in this data file were called counties.

Command

click Analyze. . . .Complex Samples. . . . Select a sample. . . . click Design a sample, click Browse: select a map and enter a name, e.g., healthscore_cs.csplan. . . .click Next. . . .Stratify by: select county. . . .Clusters: select township. . . .click Next. . .Type: Simple Random Sampling. . . .click Without replacement. . . .click Next. . . .Units: enter Counts. . . .click Value: enter 4. . . .click Next. . . .click Next. . . .click (Yes, add stage 2 now). . . .click Next. . .Stratify by: enter neighbourhood. . . .next. . .Type: Simple random sampling. . . .click Without replacement. . . .click Next. . . .Units: enter proportions. . . .click Value: enter 0,25. . . .click Next. . . .click Next. . . .click (No, do not add another stage now). . . .click Next. . .Do you want to draw a sample: click Yes. . . .Click Custom value. . . .enter 123. . . .click Next. . . .click External file, click Browse: select a map and enter a name, e.g., healthscores_cssample . . . .click Save. . . .click Next. . . .click Finish.

In the output table a summary of the sampling plan is given. In the original data file the weights of 1006 randomly sampled individuals are given. These had to be used for further analyses, and additional information on current health scores of these individuals had to be obtained and included in the cs sample file. In the maps selected above we find two new files, (1) entitled "healthscore_cs.csplan" containing the weighting procedures (this map can not be opened, but it can in closed form be entered whenever needed during further complex samples analyses of these data), and (2) entitled "healthscores_cssample" containing 1006 randomly selected individuals from the main data file. The latter data file is first completed with current health scores before the definitive analysis. Only of 974 individuals the current information could be obtained, and these data were added as a new variable (see "healthscores_cssample" at extras.springer.com). Also the file (1) has for convenience been made available at extras.springer.com.

4.3 Traditional Efficacy Analysis

We will start with a traditional analysis of the above data file (1). Open it in your computer with SPSS statistical software with the module Complex Samples included.

Command

Analyze….Descriptive Statistics….Explore….Dependent List: enter last and curhealthscores….Factor List: enter County….click Statistics….mark: Descriptives….click OK.

In the output the underneath table is given.

			Estimate	95% confidence interval
Eastern	mean	last	19,3013	19,0373-19,5653
		cur	24,5651	23,7960-25,3452
Southern		last	17,669	17,2885-18,0512
		cur	24,6023	23,7761-25,4285
Western		last	11,7100	11,3559-12,0642
		cur	14,9553	14,4485-15,4620
Northern		last	10,1281	9,8899-10,3662
		cur	15,65451	14,8993-16,3908

4.4 Complex-Samples for Efficacy Analysis

We now use the above data files (1) and (2) for a Complex-Samples Analysis. The averages will be assessed and tested of

the current and prior health scores *(I)*,
their linear relationship level *(II)*,
and their ratios *(III)*.

(I) Averages of the current and prior health scores.
Open the above data file (2).

Command
Analyze. . . .Complex Samples. . . .Descriptives. . . .click Browse: select the appropriate map and enter healthscore_cs.csplan. . . .click Continue. . .Measures: enter last healthscore, enter curhealthscore. . . .Subpopulations: enter County. . . .click Statistics: mark Mean, 95% Confidence interval, Design effect. . . .click OK.

Underneath are given the means of health scores per territorial division; complex sample analysis (upper table) and traditional random sampling analysis (lower table). The complex sample means are similar to the traditional means. However, the standard errors are, substantially, larger, sometimes 3–4 times. The current scores tend to be larger than the old scores.

County			Estimate	95% Confidence Interval	
				Lower	Upper
Eastern	Mean	last healthscore	19,3040	18,9277	19,6803
		curhealthscore	24,5659	21,0591	28,0726
"Southern	Mean	last healthscore	17,6714	16,9828	18,3601
		curhealthscore	24,5764	20,8233	28,3295
"Western	Mean	last healthscore	11,8569	11,2562	12,4576
		curhealthscore	14,9585	14,4260	15,4910
Northern	Mean	last healthscore	10,1317	9,6571	10,6063
		curhealthscore	15,6330	11,7072	19,5588

			Estimate	95% confidence interval
Eastern	mean	last	19,3013	19,0373-19,5653
		cur	24,5651	23,7960-25,3452
Southern		last	17,669	17,2885-18,0512
		cur	24,6023	23,7761-25,4285
Western		last	11,7100	11,3559-12,0642
		cur	14,9553	14,4485-15,4620
Northern		last	10,1281	9,8899-10,3662
		cur	15,65451	14,8993-16,3908

The above table upper part gives the means and 95% confidence intervals. Also design effects are given (not shown). The design effects are sometimes relevant, because they are the ratios of the variances of the complex sampling method versus those of the traditional, otherwise called simple random sampling, method. In the given example the ratios are mostly 3–4, which means that the uncertainty of the complex samples methodology is 3–4 times larger than that of the traditional method. However, this reduction in precision is compensated for by the removal of biases due to the use of inappropriate probabilities used in the traditional method.

It is remarkable to observe, that, although the two methods produce, virtually, the same means, the confidence intervals are very different. E.g., for the Northern region, curhealthscores), the 95% confidence intervals went from 11.7–19.6 to 14.9–16.4, which means, that the complex samples results estimates were about three times wider.

(II) Linear relationship level between the current and prior health scores.
Open the data file (2).

Command
Analyze. . . .Complex Samples. . . .General Linear Model. . . .click Browse: select the appropriate map and enter healthscore_cs.csplan. . . .click Continue. . .Dependent variable: enter curhealthscore. . . .Covariates: enter last healthscores. . . .click Statistics: mark Estimates, 95% Confidence interval, t-test. . . .click OK.

It may take a few seconds. The underneath table upper part gives the correlation coefficient and the 95% confidence intervals. The lower part gives the simple random sampling data obtained through the usual commands (Analyze, Regression, Linear, Dependent (curhealthscore), Independent (s) (last healthscore), OK). It is remarkable to observe the differences between the two analyses. The correlation coefficients are largely the same but their standard errors are respectively 0.158 and 0.044. The t-value of the complex sampling analysis equals 5.315, while that of the traditional analysis equals no less than 19.635. Nonetheless, the reduced precision of the complex sampling analysis did not produce a statistically insignificant result, and, in addition, it was, of course, again adjusted for inappropriate probability estimates. The table, thus, gives a linear regression of health scores, complex sample analysis (upper table) and traditional simple random sampling (srs) analysis (lower table). The complex-samples general linear model is given with last appraisal as independent and current appraisal as dependent variable. The old scores is a very significant predictor of the new scores

Parameter Estimates[a]

Parameter	Estimate	Std. Error	95% Confidence Interval Lower	95% Confidence Interval Upper	Hypothesis Test t	Hypothesis Test df	Hypothesis Test Sig.
(Intercept)	8,151	2,262	3,222	13,079	3,603	12,000	,004
lasthealthscore	,838	,158	,494	1,182	5,315	12,000	,000

a. Model: curhealthscore = (Intercept) + lasthealthscore

Coefficients[a]

Model		Unstandardized Coefficients B	Unstandardized Coefficients Std. Error	Standardized Coefficients Beta	t	Sig.
1	(Constant)	7,353	,677		10,856	,000
	last healthscore	,864	,044	,533	19,635	,000

a. Dependent Variable: curhealthscore

(III) Ratios of the current and prior health scores.
Open the data file (2).

Command

Analyze....Complex Samples....Ratios....click Browse: select the appropriate map and enter healthscore_cs.csplan....click Continue...Numerators: enter last curhealthscore....Denominator: enter last healthscore....Subpopulations: enter County....click Statistics:
mark Standard error, Confidence interval (enter 95%), Design effect....click Continue....click OK.

The underneath table gives the overall ratio and the ratios per county plus 95% confidence intervals. Also design effects are given. The design effects are the ratios of the variances of the complex sampling method versus that of the traditional, otherwise called simple random sampling (srs), method. In the given example the ratios are mostly 3–4, which means that the uncertainty of the complex samples methodology is 3–4 times larger than that of the traditional method. However, this reduction in precision is compensated for by the removal of biases due to the use of inappropriate probabilities used in the srs method.

Ratios 1

Numerator	Denominator	Ratio Estimate	Standard Error	95% Confidence Interval Lower	95% Confidence Interval Upper	Design Effect
curhealthscore	last healthscore	1,371	,059	1,244	1,499	17,566

Ratios 1

County	Numerator	Denominator	Ratio Estimate	Standard Error	95% Confidence Interval Lower	95% Confidence Interval Upper	Design Effect
Eastern	curhealthscore	last healthscore	1,273	,076	1,107	1,438	12,338
"Southern	curhealthscore	last healthscore	1,391	,100	1,174	1,608	21,895
"Western	curhealthscore	last healthscore	1,278	,039	1,194	1,362	1,518
Northern	curhealthscore	last healthscore	1,543	,170	1,172	1,914	15,806

The underneath table gives the srs (simple random sampling) data obtained through the usual commands (Analyze, Descriptive Statistics, Ratio, Numerator (curhealthscore), Denominator (lasthealthscore), Group Variable (County), Statistics (means, confidence intervals etc). Again the ratios of the complex samples and traditional analyses are rather similar, but the confidence intervals are very different. E.g., the 95% confidence intervals of the Northern County went from 1.172 to 1.914 in the complex-samples, and from 1.525 to 1.702 in the traditional analysis, and was thus over 3 times wider in the former analysis.

The underneath table thus gives ratios of health scores per county: complex sample analysis (upper table) and traditional simple random sampling (srs) analysis (above lower table). Ratios of scores of individuals in different parts of a region of current versus previous scores. Although the mean values were virtually similar to those from the traditional analysis, the SEs (standard errors) of the complex-sample assessments were 4–5 times the size of those from the traditional computations. The ratios given underscore the data from the former tables.

Ratio Statistics for curhealthscore / last healthscore

Group	Mean	95% Confidence Interval for Mean Lower Bound	95% Confidence Interval for Mean Upper Bound	Price Related Differential	Coefficient of Dispersion	Coefficient of Variation Median Centered
Eastern	1,282	1,241	1,323	1,007	,184	24,3%
"Southern	1,436	1,380	1,492	1,031	,266	33,4%
"Western	1,342	1,279	1,406	1,051	,271	37,7%
Northern	1,613	1,525	1,702	1,044	,374	55,7%
Overall	1,429	1,395	1,463	1,047	,285	41,8%

The confidence intervals are constructed by assuming a Normal distribution for the ratios.

In addition to the statistics given above, other complex-samples statistics are possible, and they can be equally well executed in SPSS, that is, if the data are appropriate. If you have a binary outcome variable (dichotomous) available, then logistic regression modeling will be possible, if an ordinal outcome variable (polytomous) is available, ordinal regression, if time to event information is in the data, then complex-samples Cox regression can be performed.

4.5 Discussion

Traditionally, the best information of a target population seems to be provided by the assessment of the entire population. However, this is costly and laborious, and broad data often suffer from flaws like low quality samples, missing data, and invalid data. The advantages of limited samples are summarized.

1. Reduced costs.
2. Greater speed.
3. Greater scope and deeper insight, because of highly specialized equipments.
4. Greater accuracy, also because of higher quality personnel and better training.

Traditional analysis of limited samples from heterogeneous target populations is a biased methodology, because each individual selected is given the same probability, and the spread in the data is, therefore, severely underestimated. In complex-sampling this bias is adjusted for by assigning appropriate weights to each individual included.

Another advantage is the possibility to conduct various types of regression analyses including linear, logistic and Cox proportional hazard modeling of adjusted complex sample data, and to compare the results with those of traditional analyses, and quantitatively assess the differences.

Complex-sampling has some disadvantages. First, it is, of course, less efficient than a traditional srs (sample registration system) analysis of a complex-sample, because it yields estimates of lower precision. Second, with traditional sampling prior sample size calculations enable to predict the statistical power of a study.

With complex-samples this is not impossible. However, it is pretty hard, because the power is not only depends on the magnitude of the outcome, but also on the individual weights of the outcome variables and the interactions between weights and the outcome. The best power is obtained if the variables in the population strata and the complex samples are proportional with one another, but also this may be hard to realize with random sampling. The current chapter shows, that the spread in the data with the complex sampling method was 3–4 times wider than it was with the simple random sampling method. Nonetheless, p-values were very small, like 0.0001, and one could argue that the data analyses given were somewhat overpowered, and that a (much) smaller complex sample from the target population in our example would also have been adequate for the null-hypotheses.

In this chapter traditional efficacy analysis of a population's health scores were tested against complex-samples methodology. We conclude the following.

1. Complex samples is a cost-efficient method for analyzing target populations thatare large and heterogeneously topographically distributions.
2. It is time-efficient.
3. It offers greater scope and deeper insight, because specialized equipments are feasible.
4. It offers greater accuracy, because higher quality personnel and better training are feasible.
5. Traditional analysis of limited samples from heterogeneous target populations is a biased methodology, because each individual selected is given the same probability, and the spread in the data is, therefore, generally underestimated. In complex sampling this bias is adjusted for by assigning appropriate weights to each individual included.
6. Current statistical software offers the possibility to conduct various types of regression analyses of complex samples including linear, logistic and Cox proportional hazard modeling.

In this chapter efficacy analyses of the effects of territorial divisions and of time on population health scores were assessed. Traditional efficacy analysis consisting of confidence intervals and simple linear regressions, and machine learning efficacy analysis consisting of complex-samples methodologies were tested against one another. The machine learning analyses provided better sensitivity of testing, and were more informative.

4.6 References

To readers requesting more background, theoretical and mathematical information of computations given, several textbooks complementary to the current production and written by the same authors are available:

Statistics applied to clinical studies 5th edition, 2012,
Machine learning in medicine a complete overview, 2015,
SPSS for starters and 2nd levelers 2nd edition, 2015,
Clinical data analysis on a pocket calculator 2nd edition, 2016,
Understanding clinical data analysis from published research, 2016,
Modern meta-analysis, 2017,
Regression analysis in clinical research, 2018,
Modern Bayesian statistics in clinical research, 2018.
The Analysis of Safety Data of Drug Trials, an Update, 2019.

All of them have been edited by Springer Heidelberg Germany.

Chapter 5
Bayesian-Network for Efficacy Analysis

Contents

Abstract In a 872 men double-blind placebo-controlled randomized parallel-group trial, the effect of 2 year pravastatin on the decrease of LDL cholesterol was tested, both traditionally, and with the help of machine learning.

Traditional efficacy analysis consisted of

unpaired t-test,
simple linear regressions,
multiple linear regressions.

Machine learning efficacy analysis consisted of Bayesian-networks methods.

The machine learning methods provided better sensitivity of testing, and were more informative.

Keywords Clinical trials · Traditional efficacy analysis · Machine learning efficacy analysis · Bayesian-networks methods

5.1 Introduction

Traditional efficacy analyses of clinical trials may consist of unpaired or paired t-tests for testing the significance of difference between the outcome of one treatment versus another. The analysis is sometimes accompanied by a regression analysis with adjustments for baseline laboratory values for improving precision. Also a traditional secondary endpoint efficacy analysis may be included.

T. J. Cleophas, A. H. Zwinderman, *Efficacy Analysis in Clinical Trials an Update*,
https://doi.org/10.1007/978-3-030-19918-0_5

Machine learning works differently, instead of means and standard deviations, proximities and patterns of data are used. Bayesian networks is another machine learning tool, that works with probabilistic graphical structures, where nodes are used to represent random variables and edges are the probabilistic dependencies between two variables. The dependencies may be expressed in the form of standardized regression coefficients, and Bayesian networks are chosen based on best fit AICs (Akaike or Bayesian information criteria which are subtractions of observed regression coefficients and likelihood measures). This may sound complex, but it works fine. In this chapter, of a placebo-controlled double-blind trial, the traditional statistical analysis will be tested against a machine learning methodology entitled Bayesian networks. The traditional efficacy analysis will consist of t-tests, and baseline adjusted multiple regression analysis.

5.2 Data Example

The data example comes from a double blind randomized parallel group clinical trial that evaluated efficacy of pravastatin to reduce cardiovascular events, and to reduce the decrease of the diameter of coronary vessels (Jukema et al, Circulation 1995; 91: 2528). The trial consisted of a random sample of 872 men with cardiovascular heart disease and normal to moderately enhanced LDL-cholesterol levels. Patients were randomized between 20 mg pravastatin DD or placebo for 2 years. Outcome variables were the change in mean diameter of the coronary segments measured at baseline and after 2 years with coronary angiography, and occurrence of coronary events during follow-up (death, myocardial infarction, stroke, coronary intervention). Four hundred thirty eight patients were randomized to pravastatin treatment and 434 to placebo. The main baseline characteristics are underneath.

	Placebo(n =434)	**Pravast (n = 438)**	**P - value**
Age (yrs): mean (SD)	56 (8)	57 (8)	0.26
LDL-cholesterol level at baseline (mmol/L): mean (SD)	4.31 (0.78)	4.30 (0.78)	0.75
HDL-cholesterol level at baseline(mmol/L): mean (SD)	0.93 (0.23)	0.93 (0.23)	0.72
baseline mean diameter coronary vessels (mm): mean (SD)	2.82 (0.48)	2.80 (0.46)	0.46
Smoking ever: n (%)	376 (87%)	402 (89%)	0.22
Current hypertension: n (%)	134 (31%)	112 (25%)	0.06

At baseline, there were no significant or substantial differences between the two groups with respect to age, baseline LDL- and HDL-cholesterol, smoking history, and current hypertension. Also the average diameter of the coronary vessels did not differ between the groups.

5.3 Traditional Efficacy Analysis

Traditional efficacy analysis consists of t-tests for continuous outcomes and chi-square tests for discrete outcomes. In Sect. 1.12, Chap. 1, the use of regression analyses for efficacy analyses is discussed, and in Sect. 1.13 the use of clinical trials for the assessment of causal health effects of factors other than medicines is discussed. For example, effects of interventions like angioplasties, surgeries, renal transplants etc. Many more factors can be tested in clinical trials, for example,

age factors
psychological factors
social factors
physical factors
economical factors,
and, any factor with a supposedly causal effect on health or sickness.

In the current chapter, the decrease of LDL-cholesterol after 2 years of treatment was measured in the patients on pravastatin, and compared to that of patients on placebo. The primary analysis consisted of an independent samples t-test.

	placebo	pravastatin	difference
sample size	434	438	
mean (mmol/l)	–0.04	1.23	1.27
standard deviation	0.59	0.68	standard error = 0.043

The mean difference between the effect of placebo and pravastatin was very significantly larger than 0.

Virtually the same result could be obtained by drawing the best fit data in the form of a linear regression line.

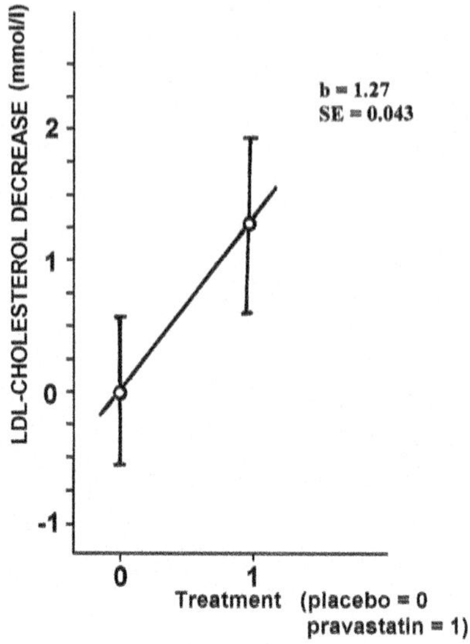

The result is very much the same as that from the above t-test with regression coefficient b and standard error (SE) equal to the mean difference between the two treatments and their pooled standard error. The advantage of regression modeling is, that better precision of the analysis can be obtained by adding a second x-variable to the regression model. Baseline LDL cholesterol was used for the purpose. The prior assumption was, that patients with high level baseline would better benefit from treatment. The linear regression model applied is given underneath.

LDL-reduction: $Y_i = \beta_0 + \beta_1 X_{1i} + e_i$ (residual error)
$X_1 =$ 1, if a patient receives pravastatin, and
zero, if he/she receives placebo
$\beta_1 =$ efficacy = 1.27 mmol/l (SE = 0.043 mmol/l, it is a function of expected standard deviation in the population (σ_e))
LDL-reduction in case of $X_1 = 1$, if a patient receives pravastatin

Suppose, there is a covariate X_2 , which is related to Y, but not to X_1.
Then, the underneath equation would be an adequate mathematical model.

$$Y_i = \beta_0 + \beta_1 X_{1i} + \beta_2 X_{2i} + e_i$$

β_1 remains the same, but σ_e^2 will be (much) smaller, and $SE_{(\beta 1)}$ will be smaller. A smaller standard error means, that the point-estimate here, being the mean decrease in LDL cholesterol, has an increased precision. An example of a variable, that might be related to Y, but not to treatment, is the baseline LDL cholesterol values. Indeed, the difference between baseline placebo and pravastatin HDL cholesterol were not significantly different from one another. Baseline LDL cholesterol is, thus, not significantly related to treatment modality in this randomized trial:

placebo: 4.32 (standard deviation (SD) 0.78)
pravastatin: 4.29 (SD 0.78),
significance level of difference between the two means p = 0.60
= 60%.

In contrast, the baseline LDL cholesterol values are very significantly linearly related to the LDL decrease.

$\beta_2 = 0.41$ (SE 0.024, $p < 0.0001$)

In addition, the efficacy parameter was equal in size, but statistically significant at a higher level:

$\beta_1 = 1.27$ (SE 0.037, was 0.043: 15% gain in efficiency).

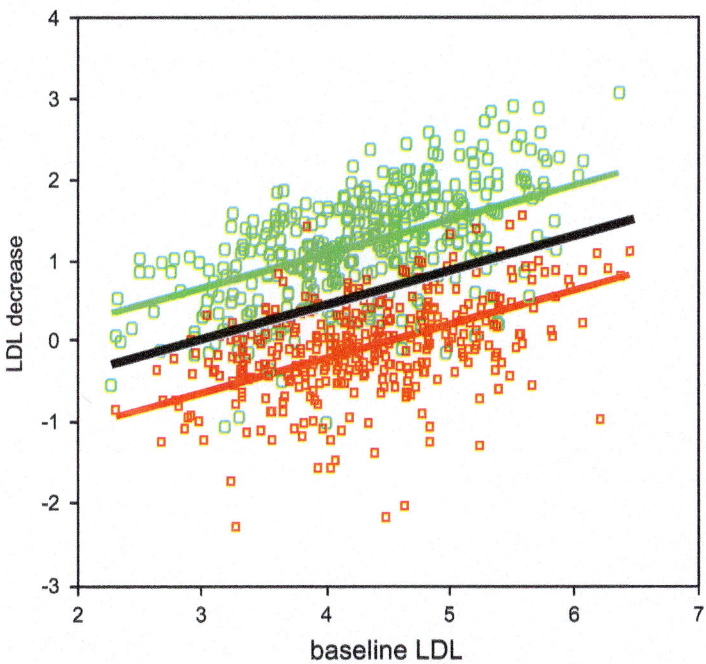

The above graph shows, that, if you replace the one regression line (black) with two novel models, then your precision will be improved. The two line model is a better fit model than the one line, and better statistics are thus obtained.

Also, secondary endpoints were included in the traditional efficacy analysis. The number of patients with a coronary events was significantly lower in the patients who were treated with pravastatin, the decrease of the diameter of the coronary vessels was also significantly lower, and the change of HDL-cholesterol levels was also significantly larger in the statin treated patients (underneath table).

	Placebo(n =434)	Pravast (n = 438)	P - value
Coronary Event: n (%)	79 (18%)	48 (11%)	0.001
Decrease of the mean diameter of the coronary vessels (mm): mean (SD)	0.10 (0.21)	0.06 (0.19)	0.014
LDL-cholesterol decrease (mmol/L): mean (SD)	-0.04 (0.59)	1.23 (0.68)	< 0.001
HDL cholesterol increase (mmol/L): mean (SD)	0.03 (0.13)	0.10 (0.16)	< 0.001

5.4 Bayesian-Network for Efficacy Analysis

Bayesian networks are probabilistic graphical models and use graphical structures to represent knowledge. In particular *nodes* and *edges* are used, where a node represents a random variable and an edge between two nodes represents a probabilistic dependency between two variables. If edges are undirected the graphical models are usually called Markov networks of Markov random fields, but in Bayesian networks edges, usually, have direction and the graph is, then, called a directed acyclic graph (DAG). With such a DAG the multivariate distribution of the variables in the DAG can be represented efficiently, and the DAG provides also an easy way to estimate the distribution.

The directed edge from variable X_i to variable X_j represents the statistical dependence of X_j and X_i, but slightly stronger, X_i is defined to influence X_j or be X_j's parent (X_j is defined to be X_i's child). In more general terms, X_j is X_i's descendant and X_i is X_j's ancestor. The DAG is acyclic and that guarantees that a variable cannot be its own descendant or ancestor. A directed edge from X_i to X_j is often understood to represent a causal relationship between the two variables X_i and X_j.

For our example data, we can consider the underneath graph of the outcome variable "coronary event: yes/no", the randomized treatment variable "pravastatin: yes/no", and the "LDL-cholesterol decrease". The directed edge between "randomized treatment" and "LDL-decrease" points to our expectation that the choice of treatment will influence how much LDL-cholesterol will decrease. The directed edge between "LDL decrease" and "coronary event" points to our expectation that the amount of LDL-decrease, in its turn, will determine the risk of a coronary event. Thus, "randomized treatment" is an ancestor of both "LDL-decrease", and "coronary event", and "LDL-decrease" is also an ancestor of "coronary event".

Bayesian networks (BNs) have rather simple conditional dependence and independence statements. The (directed) edge between "randomized treatment" and "LDL-decrease" signifies a direct dependence, namely that the distribution of the latter depends on the specific value of the former. But far more general, one may say that each variable is independent of its nondescendents in the graph given the state of its parents. Thus, "coronary event" is independent of "randomized treatment" given that the amount of "LDL-decrease" is known. Note that this particular DAG corresponds to the causal hypothesis that statin-treatment works only through lowering LDL-cholesterol level, and, thus, excludes a pleiotropic effect of statins.

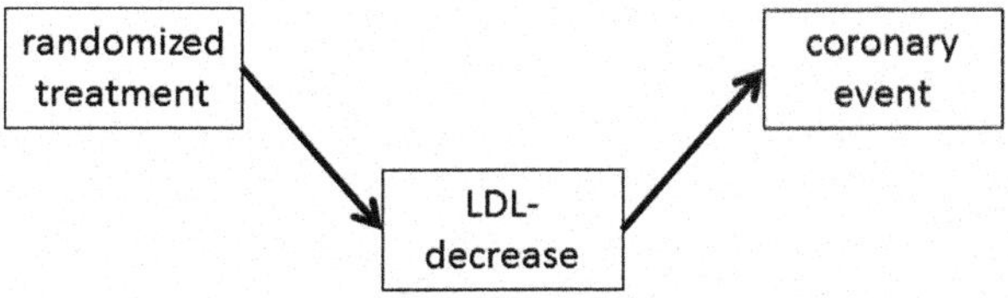

In addition to the DAG, the network is represented by a set of conditional probability distributions that together describe the multivariate distribution L(X,Y, Z) where X="randomized treatment", Y="LDL-decrease" and Z="coronary event". For the above DAG we can describe L(X,Y,Z) as the product L(X)∗L(Y|X)∗L(Z|Y), where L(Y|X) means the *likelihood* of Y given X.. Given that the randomized treatment is determined by chance, L(X) would typically be described by a Bernoulli distribution with probability 0.5 (i.e. "throwing a coin"). LDL-decrease is a normal distributed quantity and L(Y|X) would therefore be a conditional distribution usually described with ordinary linear regression and because coronary event is a binary variable L(Z|Y) would typically be described by logistic regression. Leaving out the directed edge from "randomized treatment" to "coronary event" means that L(X,Y,Z) is less complex than a saturated model, meaning that one parameter less needs to be estimated from the data. This is not very imposing, but BNs of many variables can benefit greatly from assuming structure in the sense that inference is computationally much cheaper, and results can be far more robust with far less variance. The complexity of the multivariate distribution modeled with a BN is quantified by the so-called *d-separation* statistic.

Inference in a Bayesian network is done by marginalization, meaning that irrelevant variables are integrated or summed out. If the risk of a coronary event must be calculated for patients treated with pravastatin, this is calculated by $L(Z|X{=}statin) = \int L(Z|Y{=}y)\, L(Y{=}y|X{=}statin)\, dy$. Basically, the likelihood of a coronary event for all possible LDL-decreases Y=y are considered (i.e. L(Z|Y=y)) and these likelihoods are averaged but weighted with the likelihood that such a LDL-decrease Y=y is observed under statin treatment (i.e. L(Y=y|X=statin)). For a particular variable in a general Bayesian network this marginalization can be done through either its parents or its children, and the former is called *predictive support* or *top-down reasoning* while the latter is called *diagnostic support* or *bottom-up reasoning*. Which strategy is chosen, is determined for opportunistic reasons, but if the Bayesian network is large, exact inference may be very hard involving multiple integrals or summations. Popular exact algorithms are message-passing, cycle-cutset and variable-elimination. Approximate algorithms are useful for large Bayesian networks and are mostly based on Monte Carlo sampling such as the Markov Chain Monte Carlo (MCMC) methods.

Learning a new BN from data presents several difficulties: the Bayesian network structure may be known or unknown, the shapes of the conditional distributions L $(X_j|X_i)$ and their parameters may be known or unknown, and the variables in the Bayesian network may be observed or only partially observed. Given a particular Bayesian network structure and appropriate data, the best parameters describing the multivariate distribution are found by maximization of the log-likelihood of the data. This is fully comparable to estimating any statistical model. For the Bayesian network in underneath figure this would entail estimating the parameters of the linear regression model of LDL-decrease on randomized treatment and of the logistic regression model of coronary event on LDL-decrease. If the Bayesian network contains nodes for which no data is available, then the unobserved nodes must be partialed out. This can be done using MCMC methods or with expectation-maximization algorithms in less complex cases.

If the Bayesian network structure is unknown, the problem is, unfortunately, much harder, because the number of different DAGs with N variables is superexponential in N. In practice one then, usually, starts with a reasonably simple DAG (a naive Bayesian network for instance), and, then, adds those edges to the DAG that minimize some goodness of fit criterion such as the Akaike's or Bayesian Information Criterion (AIC/BIC). This is the approach we used for our example data.

When using Matlab Bayes Net toolbox [code.google.com/p/bnt/], the following syntax commands from Matlab prompt should be given.

1. For model selection:

   `P(D|G) = \int_{\theta}p(D|G),\theta)`

2. For finding the best model:

   `\sum_{k=0}^n\choice{n}{k} = 2^n`

3. For computing BIC values:

   `\log\Pr(D|G)\approx\log\Pr(D|G).\hat{\Theta}_G) - \frac{\log N}{2} / #G`

For our data we hypothesized that the randomized treatment only affected the risk of coronary events through lowering LDL-cholesterol. We assumed that this in its turn would reduce the decrease of the diameters of the coronary vessels. We hypothesized, in addition, that smoking affects the diameters of the coronary vessels, and that hypertension has a direct effect on the risk of coronary events.

The DAG has three parents, namely "age", "smoking", and "randomized treatment". The structure also hypothesizes, that the significant association between randomized treatment and coronary events will vanish by conditioning on change of vessel diameter. Similarly, the associations between age and smoking and coronary events will vanish after conditioning on hypertension and change of vessel diameter. The AIC values of the hypothesized DAG and five adaptations are reported (table below). The optimal AIC value was found for a model in which the conditional distribution of vessel-diameter-change depended directly on smoking and randomized treatment, and that the risk of a coronary event depended on the amount of LDL- and HDL- cholesterol change, and, in addition, on the randomized treatment. This latter result may be interpreted as the pleiotropic effect of pravastatin.

The best fitting DAG was, however, much more complicated, involving dependencies between age and smoking, between smoking and baseline hypertension, LDL- and HDL-cholesterol, and of all of these on LDL- and HDL-cholesterol change and change of vessel diameter. Coronary event appeared, in contrast, to be dependent only on randomized treatment and not on LDL- or HDL-decrease. We should add, that the goodness of fit of a Bayesian network is expressed in the form of its AIC. AIC = Akaike Information Criterium = subtraction of observed regression coefficients and likelihood measures.

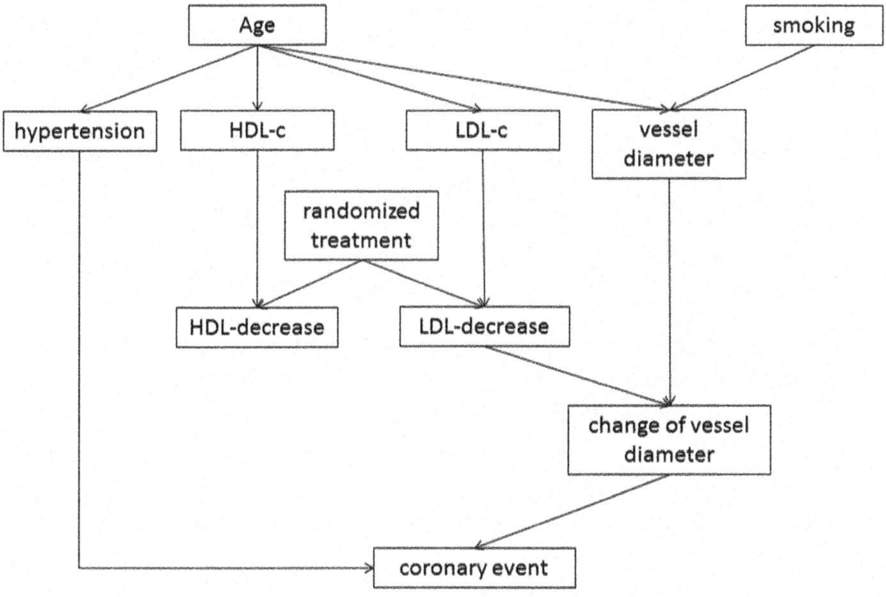

nr	model	AIC
0	as illustrated in the above figure	13147.26
1	model 0 plus direct effects of LDL- and HDL-cholesterol decreases on events	13145.15
2	model 1 plus direct effect of randomized treatment on events	13139.49
3	model 1 plus direct effect of randomized treatment on change of diameter	13143.06
4	model 2 plus direct effect of randomized treatment on change of diameter	13135.29
5	model 3 plus direct effects of smoking on events and change of diameter	13136.83

5.5 Discussion

Bayesian networks (BNs) have attained much enthusiasm in many applied research fields. The graphical interface has proved to be very helpful both in summarizing relationships between a large set of variables and for hypothesizing about causality. The graphical display has been adopted very widely, for instance, by biomolecular scientists to describe pathogenic and metabolic pathways. But the graphical tools have proved to be appealing in every applied field. The causal interpretation of BNs is (in contrast) somewhat problematic in biomedicine. Causality is difficult in biomedical research, because, often, confounding effects can not be ruled out in observational data, and it is very difficult to specify the influence of selection processes for any given sample of patients. It is also difficult to do controlled experiments with human subjects.

Aside from interpretations, BNs are very efficient to describe multivariate distributions. The structure makes inference of BNs often robust and it also reduces variance of estimated parameters. Thus BNs are often robust against overfitting. In case a new network is learned from a dataset, it is nevertheless highly recommended to perform some form of cross validation to assess reliability of the network.

Software for Bayesian networks are available in many computer programs. Several packages are available in the freeware/shareware R system [www.r-project.org, package: deal], several algorithms are offered in the weka package [weka.sourceforce.net] and the Matlab Bayes Net toolbox [code.google.com/p/bnt/].

In this chapter of a placebo-controlled double-blind trial, the traditional statistical analysis with t-test and baseline adjusted multiple regression analysis were tested against a Bayesian networks analysis.

We conclude.

1. The graphical display of Bayesian networks has been adopted very widely, for instance, by biomolecular scientists to describe pathogenic and metabolic pathways.
2. The graphical tools have proved to be appealing in every applied field. The causal interpretation of BNs is (in contrast) somewhat problematic in biomedicine.
3. Causality is difficult in biomedical research, because, often, confounding effects can not be ruled out in observational data, and it is also difficult to do controlled experiments with human subjects.
4. Bayesian networks are very efficient to describe multivariate distributions. The structure makes inferences from Bayesian networks robust, reduces variances of estimated parameters, and is also robust against overfitting.
5. Unlike traditional efficacy analyses with t-test and linear regression, Bayesian networks does not provide p-values. In contrast, relevant pathogenic and metabolic pathways can be inferenced with different levels of data fit.

In this chapter the traditional efficacy analysis consisted of unpaired t-test, simple linear regression, and multiple linear regression, and the machine learning analyses included Bayesian network methodologies. The machine learning analyses provided better sensitivity of testing, and were more informative.

5.6 References

To readers requesting more background, theoretical and mathematical information of computations given, several textbooks complementary to the current production and also written by the same authors are available:

Statistics applied to clinical studies 5th edition, 2012,
Machine learning in medicine a complete overview, 2015,
SPSS for starters and 2nd levelers 2nd edition, 2015,
Clinical data analysis on a pocket calculator 2nd edition, 2016,
Understanding clinical data analysis from published research, 2016,
Modern meta-analysis, 2017,
Regression analysis in clinical research, 2018,
Modern Bayesian statistics in clinical research, 2018.
The Analysis of Safety Data of Drug Trials, an Update, 2019.

All of them have been edited by Springer Heidelberg Germany.

Chapter 6
Evolutionary-Operations for Efficacy Analysis

Contents

Abstract In 16 operation settings, the effects of humidity, filter capacity, and air volume change on numbers of infections were tested, both traditionally, and with the help of machine learning.

Traditional efficacy analysis was composed of

Poisson statistics,

z-tests.

Machine learning efficacy analysis was composed of evolutionary-operation methods.

The machine learning methods provided better sensitivity of testing, and were more informative.

Keywords Clinical trials · Traditional efficacy analysis · Machine learning efficacy analysis · Evolutionary-operation methods

6.1 Introduction

In controlled trials continuous or binary variables are generally used for efficacy analysis. However, rates can also be applied as efficacy estimator. In this chapter traditional and machine learning efficacy analysis will be tested against one another. Traditional efficacy analysis will be done with z-statistics. Evolutionary-operations will be used as machine learning method for efficacy analysis.

T. J. Cleophas, A. H. Zwinderman, *Efficacy Analysis in Clinical Trials an Update*,
https://doi.org/10.1007/978-3-030-19918-0_6

Evolutionary operations (evops) try and find improved processes by exploring the effect of small changes in an experimental setting. It stems from evolutionary algorithms, which uses rules based on biological evolution mechanisms where each next generation is slightly different and generally somewhat improved as compared to its ancestors. It is widely used not only in genetic research, but also in chemical and technical processes. So much so that the internet nowadays offers free evop calculators suitable not only for the optimization of the above processes, but also for the optimization of your pet' s food, your car costs, and many other daily life standard issues. This chapter is to assess how evops can be used as an alternative and more sensitive method for efficacy analysis of clinical trials. The efficacy analysis will consist of Poisson statistics, z-tests.

6.2 Data Example

The air quality of operation rooms is important for infection prevention. Particularly, the factors (1) humidity (30–60%), (2) filter capacity (70–90%), and (3) air volume change (20–30% per hour) are supposed to be important determinants. The primary scientific question was: can an evolutionary operation be used for process improvement. The effect of different operation room air settings on the infection rates were studied. Underneath an overview is given of the entire data with 16 different settings.

Operation Setting	humidity (30% = 1, 60% = 4)	filter capacity (70% = 1, 90% = 3)	air volume change (20% = 1, 30% = 3)	infections number of
1	1	1	1	99
2	2	1	1	90
3	1	2	1	75
4	2	2	1	73
5	1	1	2	99
6	2	1	2	99
7	1	2	2	61
8	2	2	2	52
9	2	2	2	51
10	3	2	2	45
11	2	3	2	33
12	3	3	2	26
13	2	2	3	73
14	3	2	3	60
15	2	3	3	54
16	3	3	3	31

6.3 Traditional Efficacy Analysis

In 6 parallel-group trials the effect of two different operation room air condition settings were compared with one another. The outcome was the rate of infections per setting. Rates or proportions can be described as the probability of the corresponding outcome. For example, if the rate of infections per time and place is given, then Poisson statistics will be adequate.

The standard error (se) of rate is approached by

$$se = \sqrt{\text{rate}},$$

and z -statistic may be applied for finding p-values. A significance of difference between two rates is tested as follows.

$$z = (\text{rate } 1 - \text{rate } 2) / \sqrt{(\text{rate } 1 + \text{rate } 2)}.$$

$z > 1.96$ corresponds to a p-value of < 0.05.

Study 1

Operation Setting	humidity (30% = 1, 60% = 4)	filter capacity (70% = 1, 90% = 3)	air volume change (20% = 1, 30% = 3)	infections number of
1	1	1	1	99
2	2	1	1	90

z = (rate 1 - rate 2) / √ (rate 1 + rate 2) = (99 - 90)/√ (99+90) = 0.66
z < 1.96, p > 0.05

Study 2

Operation Setting	humidity (30% = 1, 60% = 4)	filter capacity (70% = 1, 90% = 3)	air volume change (20% = 1, 30% = 3)	infections number of
2	2	1	1	90
4	2	2	1	73

z = (rate 1 - rate 2) / √ (rate 1 + rate 2) = (90 - 73)/√ (90+73) = 1.33
z < 1.96, p > 0.05

Study 3

Operation Setting	humidity (30% = 1, 60% = 4)	filter capacity (70% = 1, 90% = 3)	air volume change (20% = 1, 30% = 3)	infections number of
4	2	2	1	73
8	2	2	2	52

z = (rate 1 - rate 2) / √ (rate 1 + rate 2) = (73-52)/√ (70+52) = 21/11= 1.91
z < 1.96, p > 0.05

Study 4

Operation Setting	humidity (30% = 1, 60% = 4)	filter capacity (70% = 1, 90% = 3)	air volume change (20% = 1, 30% = 3)	infections number of
9	2	2	2	51
10	3	2	2	45

z = (rate 1 - rate 2) / √ (rate 1 + rate 2) = (51-45)/√ (51+45) = 0.61
z < 1.96, p > 0.05

Study 5

Operation Setting	humidity (30% = 1, 60% = 4)	filter capacity (70% = 1, 90% = 3)	air volume change (20% = 1, 30% = 3)	infections number of
10	3	2	2	45
12	3	3	2	26

z = (rate 1 - rate 2) / √ (rate 1 + rate 2) = (45 - 26)/√ (45+26) = 2.26
z > 1.96, p < 0.05

Study 6

Operation Setting	humidity (30% = 1, 60% = 4)	filter capacity (70% = 1, 90% = 3)	air volume change (20% = 1, 30% = 3)	infections number of
12	3	3	2	26
16	3	3	3	31

z = (rate 1 - rate 2) / √ (rate 1 + rate 2) = (26 - 31)/√ (26+31) = -0.66
z > -1.96, p > 0.05

Except for the study 5, none of the studies produced a significant result. The setting 12 performed significantly better than the setting 10 did. However, the difference between the setting 12 and a subsequent higher level setting 16 was not significant anymore. Five of the six parallel group studies produced statistically insignificant results, and the results from them were, thus, negative. These studies were unable to reject their null-hypotheses, and demonstrate the presence of improved processes by small changes in experimental settings of operation room air condition.

6.4 Evolutionary-Operations for Efficacy Analysis

Eight operation room air condition settings were first investigated, and the results are underneath.

Operation Setting	humidity (30% = 1, 60% = 4)	filter capacity (70% = 1, 90% = 3)	air volume change (20% = 1, 30% = 3)	infections number of
1	1	1	1	99
2	2	1	1	90
3	1	2	1	75
4	2	2	1	73
5	1	1	2	99
6	2	1	2	99
7	1	2	2	61
8	2	2	2	52

We will use multiple linear regression in SPSS with the number of infections as outcome and the three factors as predictors to identify the significant predictors.

The data file available as "evops" in extras.springer.com is opened in SPSS (Var = variable).

Command

Analyze....Regression....Linear....Dependent: enter "Var00004".... Independent(s): enter "Var00001-00003)"....click OK.

The underneath table in the output shows that all of the determinants are statistically significant at $p < 0.10$. A higher humidity, filtering level, and air volume change better prevents infections.

Coefficients[a]

Model		Unstandardized Coefficients		Standardized Coefficients	t	Sig.
		B	Std. Error	Beta		
1	(Constant)	103,250	18,243		5,660	,005
	hunidity1	-12,250	3,649	-,408	-3,357	,028
	filter capacity1	-21,250	3,649	-,707	-5,824	,004
	airvolume change1	15,750	3,649	,524	4,317	,012

a. Dependent Variable: infections1

In the next 8 operation settings higher determinant levels were assessed.

Operation Setting	humidity (30% = 1, 60% = 4)	filter capacity (70% = 1, 90% = 3)	air volume change (20% = 1, 30% = 3)	infections number of
9	2	2	2	51
10	3	2	2	45
11	2	3	2	33
12	3	3	2	26
13	2	2	3	73
14	3	2	3	60
15	2	3	3	54
16	3	3	3	31

We will use again multiple linear regression in SPSS with the number of infections as outcome and the three factors as predictors to identify the significant predictors.

Command

Analyze....Regression....Linear....Dependent: enter "Var00008".... Independent(s): enter "Var00005-00007)"....click OK.

Coefficients[a]

Model		Unstandardized Coefficients		Standardized Coefficients	t	Sig.
		B	Std. Error	Beta		
1	(Constant)	145,500	15,512		9,380	,001
	humidity2	-5,000	5,863	-,145	-,853	,442
	filter capacity2	-31,500	5,863	-,910	-5,373	,006
	airvolume change2	-6,500	5,863	-,188	-1,109	,330

a. Dependent Variable: infections2

The above table in the output shows that only Var 00006 (the filter capacity) is still statistically significant. Filter capacity 3 performs better than 2, while humidity levels and air volume changes were not significantly different. We could go one step further to find out how higher levels would perform, but for now we will conclude that humidity level 2–3, filter capacity level 3, and air flow change level 2–3 are efficacious level combinations. Higher levels of humidity and air flow change is not meaningful. An additional benefit of a higher level of filter capacity cannot be excluded, but requires additional testing.

6.5 Discussion

Evolutionary operations can be used to improve the process of air quality maintenance in operation rooms. This methodology can similarly be applied for finding the best settings for numerous clinical, and laboratory settings. We have to add, that interaction between the predictors was not taken into account in the current example. For a meaningful assessment of 2- and 3-factor interactions larger samples would be required. Moreover, we have clinical arguments, that no important interactions are to be expected. The difference with the traditional efficacy analysis is, that all possible comparisons are systematically assessed, not just a few.

In this chapter the traditional efficacy analysis consisted of Poisson statistics with z-tests, and the machine learning analyses included evolutionary operations methodologies. The machine learning analyses provided better sensitivity of testing, and were more informative.

6.6 References

To readers requesting more background, theoretical and mathematical information of computations given, several textbooks complementary to the current production and written by the same authors are available:

Statistics applied to clinical studies 5th edition, 2012,
Machine learning in medicine a complete overview, 2015,
SPSS for starters and 2nd levelers 2nd edition, 2015,
Clinical data analysis on a pocket calculator 2nd edition, 2016,
Understanding clinical data analysis from published research, 2016,
Modern meta-analysis, 2017,
Regression analysis in clinical research, 2018,
Modern Bayesian statistics in clinical research, 2018.
The Analysis of Safety Data of Drug Trials, an Update, 2019.

All of them have been edited by Springer Heidelberg Germany.

Chapter 7
Automatic-Newton-Modeling for Efficacy Analysis

Contents

Abstract In two pharmaco-kinetic-and-dynamic (PKD) studies the effects of drug dosages on clinical effectiveness, and of time on plasma concentrations were tested, both traditionally, and with the help of machine learning.

Traditional efficacy analysis consisted of

linearized model of hyperbola function,

regression model of exponential function.

Machine learning efficacy analysis consisted of automatic-Newton modeling.

The machine learning methods provided better sensitivity of testing, and were more informative.

Keywords Clinical trials · Traditional efficacy analysis · Machine learning efficacy analysis · Automatic-Newton-modeling

7.1 Introduction

Pharmaco-kinetic-and-dynamic (PKD) studies like dose-effectiveness and time-concentration studies are traditionally analyzed using the algebraic properties of respectively a hyperbolic and an exponential relationship between predictor and outcome. The data are used to find the best fit parameters. Instead, for the same purpose a more modern machine learning method is possible named Automatic –

T. J. Cleophas, A. H. Zwinderman, *Efficacy Analysis in Clinical Trials an Update*,
https://doi.org/10.1007/978-3-030-19918-0_7

Newton – Modeling. In this chapter examples of PKD studies are analyzed both traditionally using their algebraic properties, and with machine learning using automatic Newton modeling. A traditional efficacy analysis will be tested against the machine learning methodology entitled automatic Newton modeling. The traditional efficacy analysis will consist of a linearized model of a hyperbola function, and a regression model of an exponential function.

7.2 Traditional Efficacy Analysis

7.2.1 Dose-Effectiveness Study

The underneath data are from a dose-effectiveness study of the effect of alfentanil dose on a pain scale.

Alfentanil dose x-axis mg/m^2	effectiveness y-axis [1- pain scale]
0,10	0,1701
0,20	0,2009
0,30	0,2709
0,40	0,2648
0,50	0,3013
0,60	0,4278
0,70	0,3466
0,80	0,2663
0,90	0,3201
1,00	0,4140
1,10	0,3677
1,20	0,3476
1,30	0,3656
1,40	0,3879
1,50	0,3649

A hyperbola function fit to the above experimental data given would look like

$$y = mx/(k + x).$$

A linearized function of the above function looking like $y = mx + b$ should be rearranged:

$$y^{-1} = [mx/(k + x)]^{-1},$$

and, then, into

$$1/y = (k/m.1/x) + 1/m,$$

This function from experimental data is, traditionally, deduced by the use of

1/y and 1/x values, instead of
y and x values.

First and last x and y values			first and last 1/x and 1/y values		
0.1	and	0.41	10	and	2.44
1.50	and	0.17	0.67	and	5.88

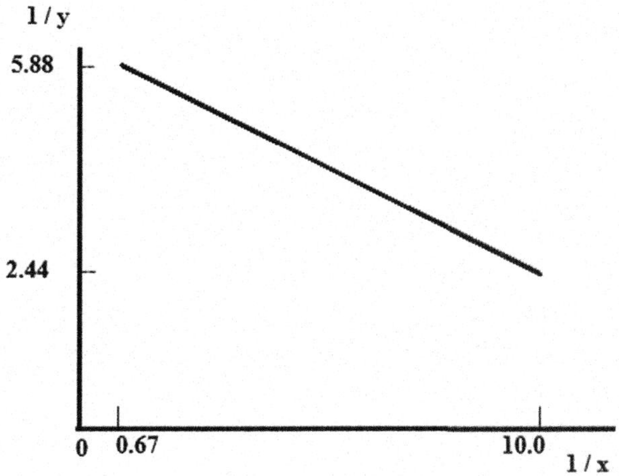

The above graph shows, that the slope of the 1/x and 1/y terms has a direction coefficient of −0.36.

Computations
2.44−5.88 = −3.44
10−0.67 = 9.33
−3.44/9.33 = −0.36.

The intercept = (5.88/9.33) times 10 = 6.30.
It equals 1/m,
m is thus 1/6.3 = 0.16,
k = −0.36 times (1/6.3) = 0.058.

Now, the equation of the hyperbola can be written

y = [0.16x/(−0.058 +x)].

7.2.2 *Time-Concentration Study*

The underneath data are from a time-concentration study of hours after quinidine administration on blood concentration.

Time x-axis hours	quinidine concentration μg/ml
0,10	0,41
0,20	0,38
0,30	0,36
0,40	0,34
0,50	0,36
0,60	0,23
0,70	0,28
0,80	0,26
0,90	0,17
1,00	0,30
1,10	0,30
1,20	0,26
1,30	0,27
1,40	0,20
1,50	0,17

The function from experimental data is, traditionally, deduced by the use of the underneath equation. The underneath key algebraic properties for an exponential trend are given.

$$F\ (x) = y = a\ b^{x}$$

$$F\ (x + \Delta x) = a\ b^{x}\ b^{x+\Delta x}$$

We will use wmueller.com.precalculusfamilies as a help.

x	y	
0.10	0.41	↓ 0.38/0.41 = 0.93
0.20	0.38	↓ 0.36/0.38 = 0.94
0.30	0.36	↓ 0.34/0.36 = 0.94
0.40	0.34	

.
.
.

$f(0.10) = a = 0.41$
With $\Delta x = 0.10$
$b^{\Delta x} = 0.94$
$b = 0.94^{1/0.1} = 0.54.$
$f(x) = 0.41.\ 0.54^{x}$

Now, the equation of an exponential function can be written (t = time in hours).

$$f(t) = 0.41.0.54^{t}.$$

7.3 Automatic-Newton-Modeling for Efficacy Analysis

Traditional regression analysis selects a mathematical function, and, then, uses the data to find the best fit parameters. For example, the parameters a and b for a linear regression function with the equation $y = a + bx$ have to be calculated according to

$$b = \text{regression coefficient} = \frac{\sum (x-\bar{x})(y-\bar{y})}{\sum (x-\bar{x})^2}$$

$$a = \text{intercept} = \bar{y} - b\bar{x}$$

With a quadratic function, $y = a + b_1x + b_2x^2$ (and other functions) the calculations are similar, but more complex. Newton's method works differently. Instead of selecting a mathematical function and using the data for finding the best fit parameter-values, it uses arbitrary parameter-values for a, b_1, b_2, and, then, iteratively measures the distance between the data and the modeled curve until the shortest distance is obtained. Calculations are much more easy than those of traditional regression analysis, making the method, particularly, interesting for comparing multiple functions to one data set. Newton's methods are mainly used for computer solutions of engineering problems, but is little used in clinical research. This chapter was to assess, whether it is also suitable for efficacy analysis of clinical trials, particularly PKD trials. We will try and answer, if these Newton's methods provide appropriate mathematical functions for dose-effectiveness and time-concentration studies. The previously used examples will be applied once again.

7.3.1 Dose-Effectiveness Study

Alfentanil dose x-axis mg/m^2	effectiveness y-axis [1- pain scale]
0,10	0,1701
0,20	0,2009
0,30	0,2709
0,40	0,2648
0,50	0,3013
0,60	0,4278
0,70	0,3466
0,80	0,2663
0,90	0,3201
1,00	0,4140
1,10	0,3677
1,20	0,3476
1,30	0,3656
1,40	0,3879
1,50	0,3649

Newton's algorithm is performed. We will use the online Nonlinear Regression Calculator of Xuru's website (This website is made available by Xuru, the world largest business network based in Auckland CA, USA. We simply copy or paste the data of the above table into the spreadsheet given by the website, then click "allow comma as decimal separator" and click "calculate". Alternatively, the SPSS file available at extras.springer.com entitled "newtonmethod" can be opened, if SPSS is installed in your computer, and the copy and paste commands are similarly given.

Since Newton's methods can be applied to (almost) any function, most computer programs fit a given dataset to over 100 functions including Gaussians, sigmoids, ratios, sinusoids etc. For the data given 18 significantly ($P < 0.05$) fitting non-linear functions were found, the first 6 of them are shown underneath.

	Non-linear function	residual sum of squares	P value
1.	$y = 0.42\,x / (x + 0.17)$	0.023	0.003
2.	$y = -1 / (38.4\,x + 1)^{0.12} + 1$	0.024	0.003
3.	$y = 0.08 \ln x + 0.36$	0.025	0.004
4.	$y = 0.40\,e^{-0.11/x}$	0.025	0.004
5.	$y = 0.36\,x^{0.26}$	0.027	0.004
6.	$y = -0.024 / x + 0.37$	0.029	0.005

The first one gives the best fit. Its measure of certainty, given as residual sum of squares, is 0.023. It is the function of a hyperbola:

$$y = 0.42\,x/(x + 0.17).$$

This is convenient, because, dose-effectiveness curves are, often, successfully assessed with hyperbolas mimicking the Michaelis-Menten equation. The parameters of the equation can be readily interpreted as $\text{effectiveness}_{\text{maximum}} = 0.42$, and dissociation constant $= 0.17$. It is usually very laborious to obtain these parameters from traditional regression modeling of the quantal effect histograms and cumulative histograms, requiring data samples of at least 100 or so to be meaningful. The underneath figure shows an Excel graph of the fitted non-linear function for the data, using Newton's method (the best fit curve is here a hyperbola). A cubic spline goes smoothly through every point, and does this by ensuring, that the first and second derivatives of the segments match those that are adjacent.

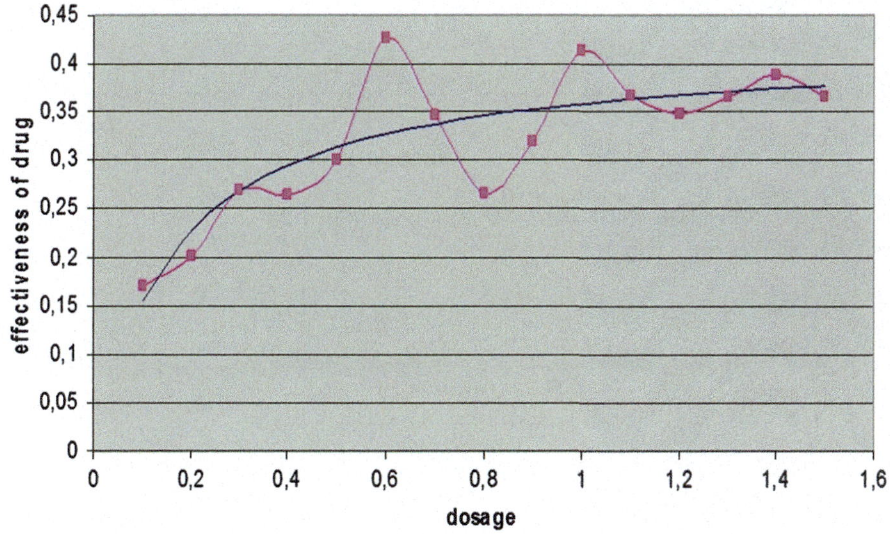

The Newton's equation better fits the data than traditional modeling with linear, logistic, quadratic, and polynomial modeling does, as shown underneath.

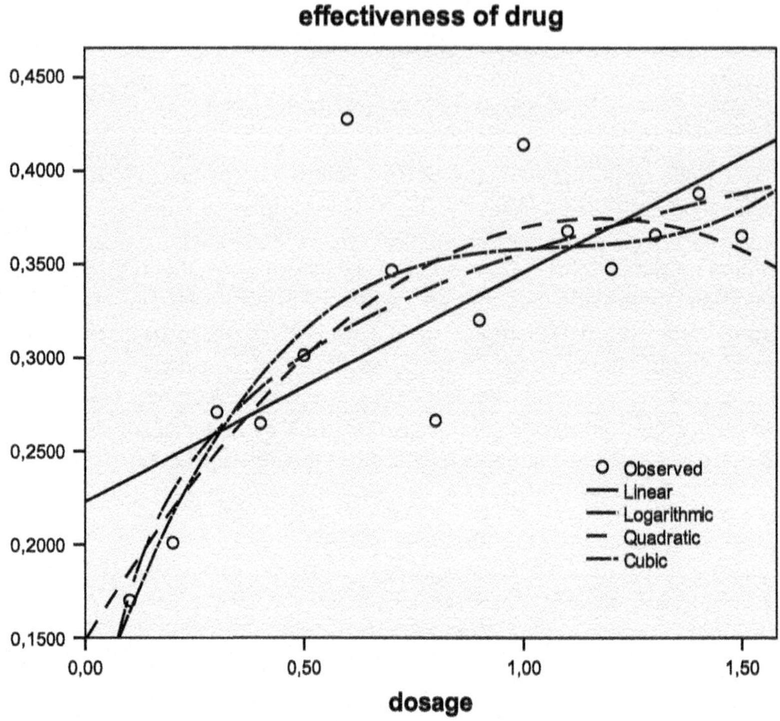

7.3.2 *Time-Concentration Study*

Time x-axis hours	quinidine concentration µg/ml
0,10	0,41
0,20	0,38
0,30	0,36
0,40	0,34
0,50	0,36
0,60	0,23
0,70	0,28
0,80	0,26
0,90	0,17
1,00	0,30
1,10	0,30
1,20	0,26
1,30	0,27
1,40	0,20
1,50	0,17

Also the above time concentration study analyzed once more, but, now, again a non-linear regression using Newton's algorithm is performed. We use the online Nonlinear Regression Calculator of Xuru's website. We copy or paste the data of the above table into the spreadsheet, then click "allow comma as decimal separator" and click "calculate". Alternatively, the SPSS file available at extras.springer.com entitled "newtonmethod" can be opened, if SPSS is installed in your computer, and the copy and paste commands are similarly given. For the data given 10 statistically significantly ($P < 0.05$) fitting non-linear functions were found and shown. For further assessment of the data an exponential function, which is among the first 5 shown by the software, is chosen, because relevant pharmacokinetic parameters can be conveniently calculated from it:

$$y = 0.41\ e^{-0.48x}.$$

This function's measure of uncertainty (residual sums of squares) value is 0.027, with a p-value of 0.003). The following pharmacokinetic parameters are derived:

$0.41 = C_0 =$ (administration dosage drug)/(distribution volume)
$-0.48 =$ elimination constant.

Below an Excel graph of the exponential function fitted to the data is given. Also, a cubic spline curve going smoothly through every point, and to be considered, as a perfect fit curve, is again given. It can be observed from the figure that the exponential function curve matches the cubic spline curve well.

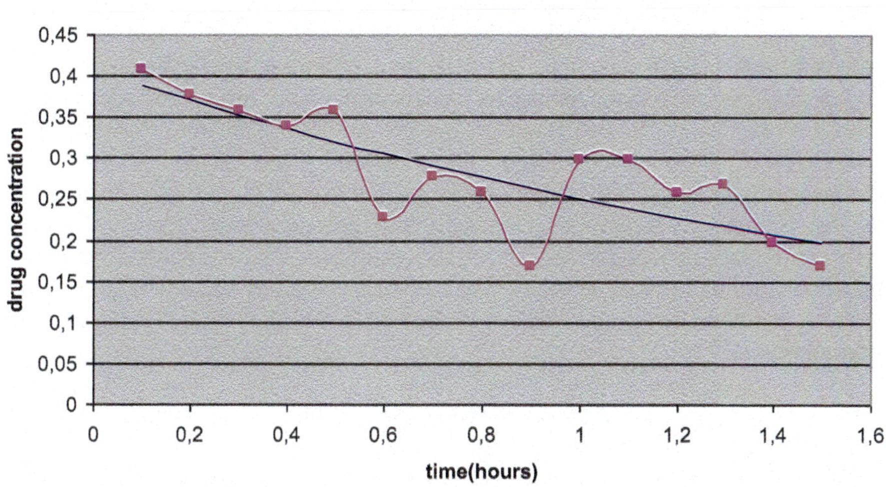

The Newton's equation fits the data approximately equally well as do traditional best fit models with linear, logistic, quadratic, and polynomial modeling shown underneath. However, traditional models do not allow for the computation of pharmacokinetic parameters.

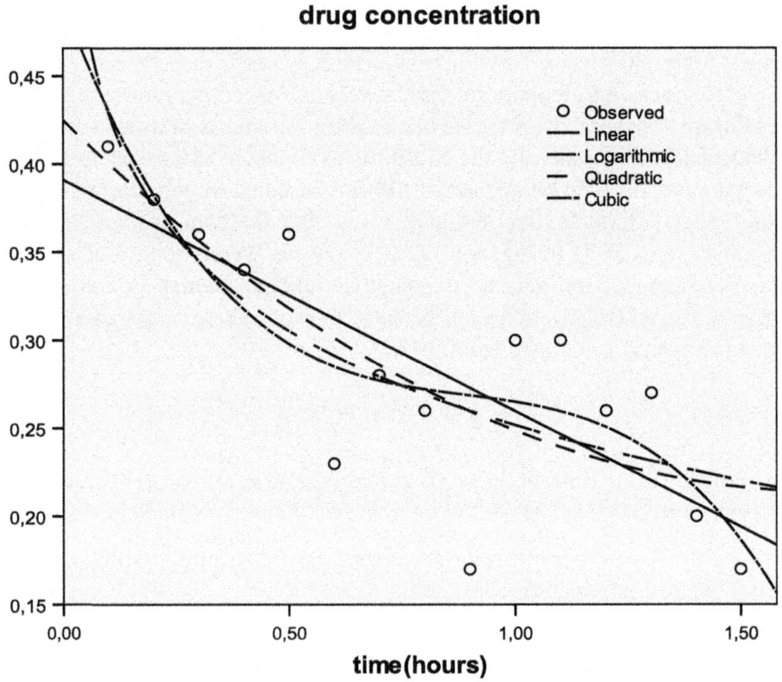

7.4 Discussion

Dose-effectiveness and time-concentration studies are, traditionally, analyzed using the algebraic properties of respectively a hyperbolic and an exponential relationship between predictor and outcome. The data are used to find the best fit parameters, which gives the best fit mathematical model for the data. Instead, a more modern machine learning method is possible, named Automatic-Newton-Modeling. The advantages of Newton's modeling is, that measures of certainty can be given. For that purpose it is statistically tested how far distant from the best fit statistical model the data actually are. Newton's methods provide appropriate mathematical functions for dose-effectiveness and time-concentration studies. In this chapter traditional and machine learning efficacy analyses were tested against one another. The machine learning method, unlike the traditional method, enabled to provide measures of uncertainty.

In this chapter the traditional efficacy analysis consisted of a linearized model of hyperbola function, and a regression model of exponential function, and the machine learning analyses included autonomic Newton modelings. The machine learning analyses provided better sensitivity of testing, and were more informative.

7.5 References

To readers requesting more background, theoretical and mathematical information of computations given, several textbooks complementary to the current production and written by the same authors are available:

Statistics applied to clinical studies 5th edition, 2012,
Machine learning in medicine a complete overview, 2015,
SPSS for starters and 2nd levelers 2nd edition, 2015,
Clinical data analysis on a pocket calculator 2nd edition, 2016,
Understanding clinical data analysis from published research, 2016,
Modern meta-analysis, 2017,
Regression analysis in clinical research, 2018,
Modern Bayesian statistics in clinical research, 2018.
The Analysis of Safety Data of Drug Trials, an Update, 2019.

All of them have been edited by Springer Heidelberg Germany.

Chapter 8
High-Risk-Bins for Efficacy Analysis

Contents

Abstract In 1445 families the effect of risk factors on overweight was tested, both traditionally and with the help of machine learning.

Traditional efficacy analysis was composed of

discretization of continuous predictors,

three dimensional bars of effects versus outcome,

crosstabs with chi-square statistics.

Machine learning efficacy analysis was composed of high-risk-bin methods.

The machine learning methods provided better sensitivity of testing, and were more informative.

Keywords Clinical trials · Traditional efficacy analysis · Machine learning efficacy analysis · High-risk-bin methods

8.1 Introduction

Risk factors of disease can be analyzed with continuous variables as predictors and the risk or odds of disease as outcome. Three-dimensional bars are helpful for visualizing data patterns and 2 × 2 crosstabs can be used for statistical testing. This traditional efficacy analysis does not provide the best fit high risk bins in your data. For that purpose some machine learning procedure is required. Particularly, optimal binning is a helpful, although pretty complex, methodology. It is a method for multi-interval discretization of continuous value intervals, and makes use of the minimum description length methodology, based on Ockham (1347) 's razor. The

T. J. Cleophas, A. H. Zwinderman, *Efficacy Analysis in Clinical Trials an Update*,
https://doi.org/10.1007/978-3-030-19918-0_8

term razor is a metaphor of the “lex parsimoniae” (latin), which tells, that, among competing hypotheses, the one with the fewest assumptions be prefered. This theory is an important concept not only in learning theory, but also in current information technology. A numerical example is given.

x =	1.0	y =	3.0
	1.3		3.3
	2.4		4.4
	3.6		5.6
	4.7		6.7

The above ten values can be described in a less lengthy way, namely

x =	1.0
	1.3
	2.4
	3.6
	4.7

and

y = x + 2

The above summary of the ten values only requires 6 instead of 10 formulations, and is, thus, considerably shorter, and, thus, more efficient to describe these data. Optimal bins describe continuous predictor variables in the form of best fit categories for making predictions, e.g., about families at high risk of bank loan defaults. In addition, it can be used for, e.g., predicting health risk cut-offs about individual future families, based on their characteristics. Can optimal binning also be applied for other medical purposes, e.g., for finding high risk cut-offs for overweight children in particular families? In this chapter a traditional efficacy analysis was tested against a machine learning efficacy analysis with high-risk-bins methodology. The traditional efficacy analysis consisted of discretized continuous predictor variables, three dimensional bars of effects versus outcomes, and crosstabs with chi-square statistics.

8.2 Traditional Efficacy Analysis

Traditional efficacy analysis consists of t-tests for continuous outcomes and chi-square tests for discrete outcomes. In Sect. 1.12, Chap. 1, the use of regression analyses for efficacy analyses is discussed, and in Sect. 1.13 the use of clinical trials for the assessment of causal health effects of factors other than medicines is discussed. For example, effects of interventions like angioplasties, surgeries, renal transplants etc. Many more factors can be tested in clinical trials, for example,

age factors
psychological factors
social factors
physical factors
economical factors,
and, any factor with a supposedly causal effect on health or sickness.

In the current chapter, in an efficacy study of 1445 families the effect of risk factors of overweight was assessed. First, the Descriptives of the predictors were computed. We will use SPSS statistical software, and the data file is in extras.springer.com, and is entitled “optimalbinning”.

Command

Analyze. . . .Descriptive Statistics. . . . Descriptives. . . .Variable(s): enter fruitvegetables/wk, unhealthysnacks/wk,fastfoodmeals/wk, physicalactivitiesd/wk. . . . click OK.

The underneath table is in the output.

Descriptive Statistics

	N	Minimum	Maximum	Mean	Std. Deviation
fruitvegetables/wk	1445	0	34	7,67	7,147
unhealthysnacks/wk	1445	0	42	10,23	6,749
fastfoodmeal/wk	1445	0	21	1,57	2,115
physicalactivities/wk	1445	0	10	7,15	2,581
Valid N (listwise)	1445				

We will use the means for cut-offs between much and little. For further assessment discretized variables will be produced with the help of the compute variable commands.

Command

Transform. . . .Compute Variable. . . .Target Variable: enter term "fruit". . . .Numeric Expression: enter variable fruitvegetables/wk. . . .click from diagram below ">". . . . click "8". . . .click OK.

In the Data View screen of your computer a binary variable entitled "fruit" is now present.

Perform the same procedure also for the unhealthysnacks, fastfood and physicalactivities variables with cut-offs for discretization >10, >2, >7. In the end we will have 4 novel variables, that can be used for traditional efficacy assessments. First, 3-D Bars will be computed, and they will display bars with few families as well as bars with lot of fruit.

Command

Graphs....Legacy Dialogs....3-D Bars....mark Groups of Cases....click Define....X Category Axis: enter the novel variable "fruit"....Z Category Axis: enter variable overweight children....click OK.

In the output it is shown, that with 3-D Bars a qualitative assessment is very well possible.

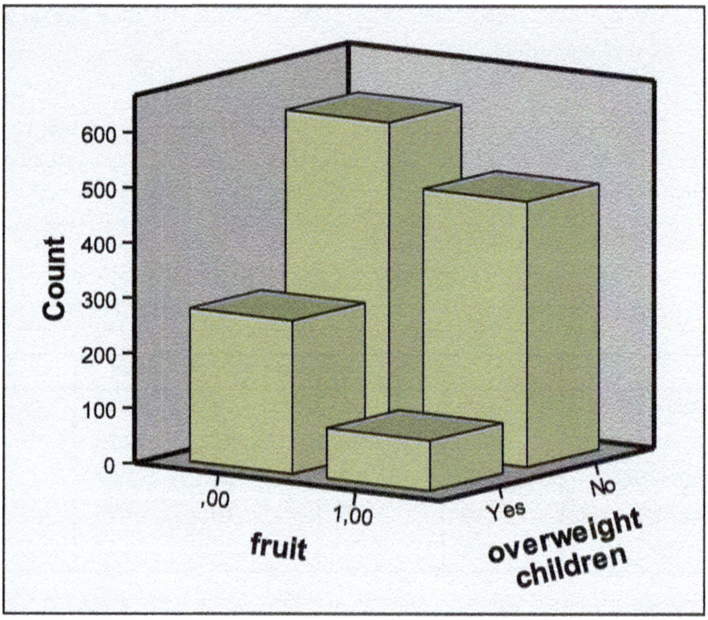

Obviously, very few families with lot of fruit intake have overweight children.

The same procedure is followed for the other three novel variables. The outputs are underneath.

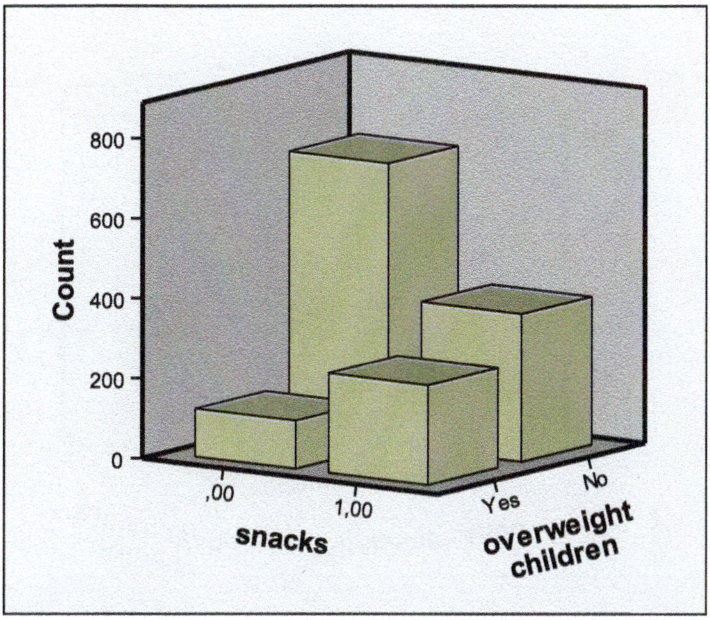

Very few families have few snacks and overweight.

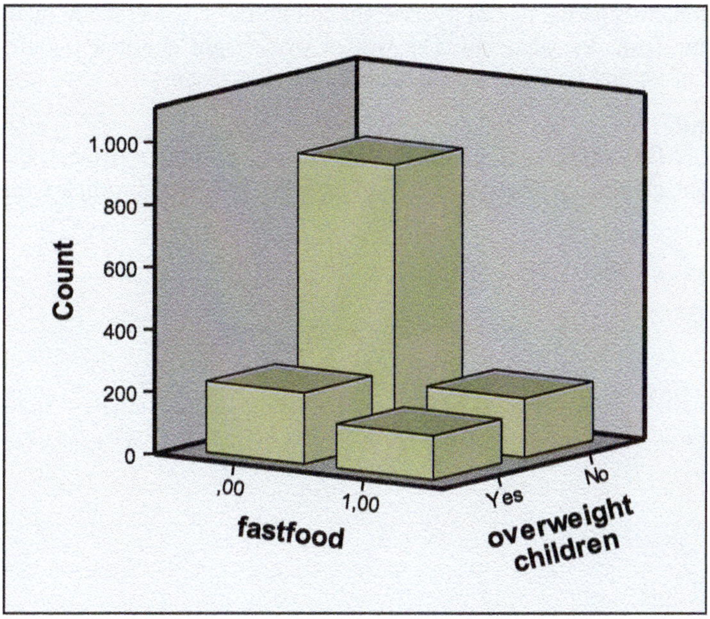

Very many families do not eat fastfood and have no overweight.

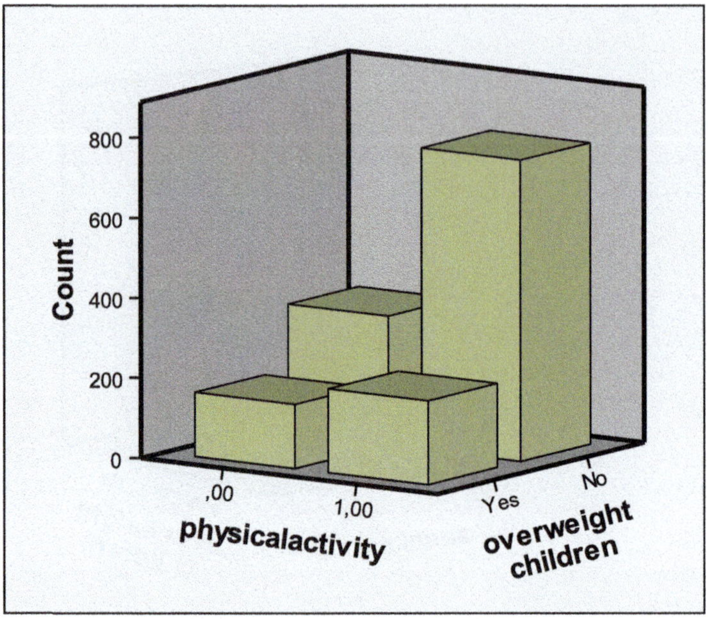

Very many families do a lot of physical activities and have no overweight.

In order to statistically test the significance of difference between the effect of the binary predictors on the risk of overweight children 2 × 2 interaction matrices with Chi-square Tests are adequate. The risk of overweight children is outcome, the presence of lot and few risk factors are used parallel groups.

Command

Analyze....Descriptive Statistics....Crosstabs....Row(s): fruit....Column(s): overweight children....Statistics....mark: click Chi-square....click Continue.... click OK.

The fruit table is in the output.

The Fruit table

Chi-Square Tests

	Value	df	Asymp. Sig. (2-sided)	Exact Sig. (2-sided)	Exact Sig. (1-sided)
Pearson Chi-Square	46,549[a]	1	,000		
Continuity Correction[b]	45,711	1	,000		
Likelihood Ratio	48,669	1	,000		
Fisher's Exact Test				,000	,000
Linear-by-Linear Association	46,517	1	,000		
N of Valid Cases	1445				

a. 0 cells (,0%) have expected count less than 5. The minimum expected count is 146,32.
b. Computed only for a 2x2 table

Also the other three binary predictors are tested similarly. The tables are given.
The Snacks table

Chi-Square Tests

	Value	df	Asymp. Sig. (2-sided)	Exact Sig. (2-sided)	Exact Sig. (1-sided)
Pearson Chi-Square	122,888[a]	1	,000		
Continuity Correction[b]	121,540	1	,000		
Likelihood Ratio	123,006	1	,000		
Fisher's Exact Test				,000	,000
Linear-by-Linear Association	122,803	1	,000		
N of Valid Cases	1445				

a. 0 cells (,0%) have expected count less than 5. The minimum expected count is 158,07.
b. Computed only for a 2x2 table

The Fastfood table

Chi-Square Tests

	Value	df	Asymp. Sig. (2-sided)	Exact Sig. (2-sided)	Exact Sig. (1-sided)
Pearson Chi-Square	66,467[a]	1	,000		
Continuity Correction[b]	65,300	1	,000		
Likelihood Ratio	61,865	1	,000		
Fisher's Exact Test				,000	,000
Linear-by-Linear Association	66,421	1	,000		
N of Valid Cases	1445				

a. 0 cells (,0%) have expected count less than 5. The minimum expected count is 84,27.
b. Computed only for a 2x2 table

The Physicalactivities table

Chi-Square Tests

	Value	df	Asymp. Sig. (2-sided)	Exact Sig. (2-sided)	Exact Sig. (1-sided)
Pearson Chi-Square	21,979[a]	1	,000		
Continuity Correction[b]	21,384	1	,000		
Likelihood Ratio	21,433	1	,000		
Fisher's Exact Test				,000	,000
Linear-by-Linear Association	21,964	1	,000		
N of Valid Cases	1445				

a. 0 cells (,0%) have expected count less than 5. The minimum expected count is 123,34.
b. Computed only for a 2x2 table

All of the above tables show very significant effects of the predictors on the outcome overweight children, but we still do not know what cut-off level between lot and little provides the best fit high risk bins of families. For that purpose a machine learning procedure is required.

8.3 High-Risk-Bins for Efficacy Analysis

Optimal bins describe continuous predictor variables in the form of best fit categories for making predictions, e.g., about families at high risk of bank loan defaults. In addition, it can be used for, e.g., predicting health risk cut-offs about individual future families, based on their characteristics. Can optimal binning also be applied for other medical purposes, e.g., for finding high risk cut-offs for overweight children in particular families?

The above used data file of 1445 families was assessed for learning the best fit cut-off values of unhealthy lifestyle estimators to maximize the difference between low and high risk of overweight children. These cut-off values were, subsequently, used to determine the risk profiles (the characteristics) in individual future families.

Var 1	Var 2	Var 3	Var 4	Var 5
0	11	1	8	0
0	7	1	9	0
1	25	7	0	1
0	11	4	5	0
1	5	1	8	1
0	10	2	8	0
0	11	1	6	0
0	7	1	8	0
0	7	0	9	0
0	15	3	0	0

Var = variable
Var 1fruitvegetables (times per week)
Var 2 unhealthysnacks (times per week)
Var 3 fastfoodmeal (times per week)
Var 4 physicalactivities (times per week)
Var 5 overweightchildren (0 = no, 1 = yes)

Only the first 10 families of the original learning data file are given, the entire data file is entitled "optimalbinning1" and is in extras.springer.com. Start by opening the data file in your computer with SPSS statistical software installed.

Command

Transform….Optimal Binning….Variables into Bins: enter fruitvegetables, unhealthysnacks, fastfoodmeal, physicalactivities….Optimize Bins with Respect to: enter "overweightchildren"….click Output….Display: mark Endpoints…. mark Descriptive statistics….mark Model Entropy….click Save: mark Create variables that contain binned data….Save Binning Rules in a Syntax file: click Browse…. open appropriate folder….File name: enter, e.g., "exportoptimalbinning"….click Save….click OK.

The underneath tables are in the output sheets.

fruitvegetables/wk

Bin	End Point		Number of Cases by Level of overweight children		
	Lower	Upper	No	Yes	Total
1	[a]	14	802	340	1142
2	14	[a]	274	29	303
Total			1076	369	1445

Each bin is computed as Lower <= fruitvegetables/wk < Upper.

a. Unbounded

unhealthysnacks/wk

Bin	End Point		Number of Cases by Level of overweight children		
	Lower	Upper	No	Yes	Total
1	[a]	12	830	143	973
2	12	19	188	126	314
3	19	[a]	58	100	158
Total			1076	369	1445

Each bin is computed as Lower <= unhealthysnacks/wk < Upper.

a. Unbounded

fastfoodmeal/wk

Bin	End Point		Number of Cases by Level of overweight children		
	Lower	Upper	No	Yes	Total
1	a	2	896	229	1125
2	2	a	180	140	320
Total			1076	369	1445

Each bin is computed as Lower <= fastfoodmeal/wk < Upper.

a. Unbounded

physicalactivities/wk

Bin	End Point		Number of Cases by Level of overweight children		
	Lower	Upper	No	Yes	Total
1	a	8	469	221	690
2	8	a	607	148	755
Total			1076	369	1445

Each bin is computed as Lower <= physicalactivities/wk < Upper.

a. Unbounded

In the output sheets, the above tables are given. It shows the high risk cut-offs for overweight children of the four predicting factors. E.g., in

1142 families scoring under 14 units of (1) fruit/vegetable per week,
are put into bin 1 and

303 scoring over 14 units per week,
are put into bin 2.

The proportion of overweight children in bin 1 is much larger than it is in bin 2:

$$340/1142 = 0.298\ (30\%)\ \text{and}\ 29/303 = 0.096\ (10\%).$$

Similarly high risk cut-offs are found for (2) unhealthy snacks less than 12, 12–19, and over 19 per week, (3) fastfood meals less than 2, and over 2 per week, (4) physical activities less than 8 and over 8 per week.

The above tables can considered a learning model for future predictions. In the current example, the cut-offs will be used as meaningful recommendation limits to eleven future families. The data of 11 future families are given underneath

fruit	snacks	fastfood	physical
13	11	4	5
2	5	3	9
12	23	9	0
17	9	6	5
2	3	3	3
10	8	4	3
15	9	3	6
9	5	3	8
2	5	2	7
9	13	5	0
28	3	3	9

Var 1fruitvegetables (times per week)
Var 2 unhealthysnacks (times per week)
Var 3 fastfoodmeal (times per week)
Var 4 physicalactivities (times per week)

The saved syntax file entitled "exportoptimalbinning" is in extras.springer.com, and will now be used to compute the predicted bins of some future families. Enter the above values in a new data file, entitled, e.g., "optimalbinning2", and save in the appropriate folder in your computer. Then open up the data file, and command.

Command
"exportoptimalbinning" ....subsequently click File....click Open....click Data.... Find the data file entitled "optimalbinning2"....click Open....click "exportoptimalbinning.sps" from the file palette at the bottom of the screen.... click Run....click All.

When returning to the Data View of "optimalbinning2", we will find the underneath overview of all of the bins selected for our eleven future families.

fruit	snacks	fastfood	physical	fruit _bin	snacks _bin	fastfood _bin	physical _bin
13	11	4	5	1	1	2	1
2	5	3	9	1	1	2	2
12	23	9	0	1	3	2	1
17	9	6	5	2	1	2	1
2	3	3	3	1	1	2	1
10	8	4	3	1	1	2	1
15	9	3	6	2	1	2	1
9	5	3	8	1	1	2	2
2	5	2	7	1	1	2	1
9	13	5	0	1	2	2	1
28	3	3	9	2	1	2	2

This overview is relevant, since families in high risk bins would particularly qualify for counseling.

8.4 Discussion

Risk factors of disease can be analyzed with continuous variables as predictors and the risk of odds of disease as outcome. Three-dimensional bars are helpful for visualizing data patterns and 2 × 2 crosstabs can be used for statistical testing. This traditional efficacy analysis does not provide the best fit high risk bins in your data. For that purpose optimal binning is a helpful, although pretty complex methodology. Optimal bins describe continuous predictor variables in the form of best fit categories for making predictions, e.g., about families at high risk of' bank loan defaults. In addition, it can be used for, e.g., predicting health risk cut-offs about individual future families, based on their characteristics. The current chapter shows, that optimal binning can be applied as a machine learning methods for efficacy analysis of clinical trials. In addition, and unlike traditional efficacy analysis, it can be used as a learning computer model for making predictions about future observations, for example, for finding high risk cut-offs for overweight children in particular families.

In this chapter the traditional efficacy analysis consisted of discretized continuous predictors, three dimensional bars of effects versus outcome, and crosstabs with chi-square statistics,and the machine learning analyses included high risk bins methodology. The machine learning analyses provided better sensitivity of testing, and were more informative.

8.5 References

To readers requesting more background, theoretical and mathematical information of computations given, several textbooks complementary to the current production and written by the same authors are available:

Statistics applied to clinical studies 5th edition, 2012,
Machine learning in medicine a complete overview, 2015,
SPSS for starters and 2nd levelers 2nd edition, 2015,
Clinical data analysis on a pocket calculator 2nd edition, 2016,
Understanding clinical data analysis from published research, 2016,
Modern meta-analysis, 2017,
Regression analysis in clinical research, 2018,
Modern Bayesian statistics in clinical research, 2018.
The Analysis of Safety Data of Drug Trials, an Update, 2019.

All of them have been edited by Springer Heidelberg Germany.

Chapter 9
Balanced-Iterative-Reducing-Hierarchy for Efficacy Analysis

Contents

Abstract In a random sample of 50 mentally depressed patients the effect of age on depression score was tested, both traditionally, and with the help of machine learning.

Traditional efficacy analysis was composed of

simple linear regressions,
discretization of continuous predictors,
multiple binary logistic regressions.

Machine learning efficacy analysis was composed of balanced-iterative-reducing-hierarchy methods.

The machine learning methods provided better sensitivity of testing, and were more informative.

Keywords Clinical trials · Traditional efficacy analysis · Machine learning efficacy analysis · Balanced-Iterative-Reducing-Hierarchy methods

9.1 Introduction

In a well-designed parallel-group trial the only difference between a treatment group and control group is the treatment. Instead of different treatment groups, sometimes other predictors are applied like different age groups, groups with different educations, races etc. One difference in a trial is of course theoretically so. In practice many differences do exist, and raise the risk of biases. Data plots are convenient for visualizing outliers in therapeutic data patterns. Outlier data are considered as

T. J. Cleophas, A. H. Zwinderman, *Efficacy Analysis in Clinical Trials an Update*,
https://doi.org/10.1007/978-3-030-19918-0_9

dependent adverse effects of the main predictor on the outcome data. They are, however, arbitrary, and, with large data files, both data pattern and outlier recognition require a more sophisticated approach. Also, the number of outliers, generally, tends to rise with the sample size. BIRCH is the abbreviation of "balanced iterative reducing hierarchies", and is available in SPSS's module Classify, under "two-step cluster analysis". The current chapter, using a simulated and a real data example, examines whether BIRCH clustering is better able than traditional efficacy analysis to detect previously unrecognized outlier data. Outliers once detected, could be removed from the data. In this chapter traditional efficacy analysis will be tested against the machine learning methodology entitled balanced iterative reducing hierarchy. Two data examples will be given. The traditional efficacy analysis will consist of simple linear regressions, discretized continuous predictors, and multiple binary logistic regressions.

9.2 Traditional Efficacy Analysis

Traditional efficacy analysis consists of t-tests for continuous outcomes and chi-square tests for discrete outcomes. In Sect. 1.12, Chap. 1, the use of regression analyses for efficacy analyses is discussed, and in Sect. 1.13 the use of clinical trials for the assessment of causal health effects of factors other than medicines is discussed. For example, effects of interventions like angioplasties, surgeries, renal transplants etc. Many more factors can be tested in clinical trials, for example,

age factors
psychological factors
social factors
physical factors
economical factors,
and, any factor with a supposedly causal effect on health or sickness.

Example 1
In patients with mental depression two classes may be identified. One with endogenous depression and one with reactive depression. Endogenous depression causes severe depression in the younger, reactive depression causes mild depression in the elderly. Age may thus predict depression scores. Insomnia is another producer of depression, and may be an outlier in a predictive study of the effects of age on depression. In a data file of 50 mentally depressed patients the effect of age on depression score was first assessed. The data file is in extras.springer.com, and is entitled "birch1".

The first 10 patients are underneath

Age Depression score
20,00 8,00
21,00 7,00
23,00 9,00
24,00 10,00
25,00 8,00
26,00 9,00
27,00 7,00
28,00 8,00
24,00 9,00
32,00 9,00

A simple linear regression with age as predictor and depression score as outcome was first performed. SPSS statistical software was applied. Start by opening the data file in your computer mounted with the software program.

Command
Analyze....Regression....Linear....Dependent: enter depressionscore....Independent(s): enter age....click OK.

The underneath table is in the output sheets.

Coefficients[a]

Model		Unstandardized Coefficients		Standardized Coefficients	t	Sig.
		B	Std. Error	Beta		
1	(Constant)	6,947	,939		7,400	,000
	age	-,033	,017	-,265	-1,903	,063

a. Dependent Variable: depressionscore

A trend to negative linear correlation is between age and depression score. In line with the above clinical argument of two age classes of depression, next the age variable was discretized in patients > and < than 40 years of age.

Command
Transform....Compute Variable....Target Variable: enter "ageclass"....Numeric Expression: enter age....from the blue diagram below add ">"....add "40".... click OK.

In the data view screen now a novel variable entitled ageclass is shown. Subsequently we will perform again a simple regression analysis with the novel variable as predictor and depression score as outcome. The underneath table is in the output sheet.

Coefficients[a]

Model		Unstandardized Coefficients		Standardized Coefficients	t	Sig.
		B	Std. Error	Beta		
1	(Constant)	6,222	,558		11,149	,000
	ageclass	-1,472	,698	-,291	-2,110	,040

a. Dependent Variable: depressionscore

A parallel-group study of two age classes of patients mental depression thus produces a significantly different effect at p = 0.04, with the younger patients more at risk than the older patients. This analysis is pretty limited, because a p-value of 0.04 is not very powerful, and a type I error can not be excluded.

Example 2

In patients admitted to hospital for iatrogenic reasons, age class was assumed to be a significant predictor of number of concomitant medications. In a 2000 patient study of hospital admissions 576 possibly iatrogenic were identified by a team of specialists. The SPSS data file is in extras.springer.com and is entitled "birch2". The number of concomitant medications (co-medications) did not significantly predict hospital admissions in the logistic model of the data, but, when transformed into a categorical predictor model, it did. Open the data file in your computer mounted with SPSS statistical software (VAR = variable).

Command

Analyze....Regression....Binary Logistic....Dependent: iatrogenic admission.... Independent: VAR00001, 00002, 00010, 00009....click OK.

The underneath table is in the output sheets. It shows the results of a multiple binary logistic regression analysis of 2000 admissions to hospital with the odds of iatrogenic admission as *dependent* variable and age (variable 00001) , gender (variable 00002), presence of co-morbidity (variable 00009, yes = 0, no = 1), and number of co-medications (variable 00010, zero to eight co-medications) as *independent* variables (p-values <0.10 are defined statistically significant).

Variables in the Equation

		B	S.E.	Wald	df	Sig.	Exp(B)
Step 1[a]	VAR00001	-,023	,004	32,062	1	,000	,977
	VAR00002	,089	,116	,580	1	,446	1,093
	VAR00010	,004	,072	,003	1	,953	1,004
	VAR00009	,095	,073	1,672	1	,196	1,099
	Constant	43,752	8,077	29,345	1	,000	1,003E19

a. Variable(s) entered on step 1: VAR00001, VAR00002, VAR00010, VAR00009.

Obviously, age is the only significant predictor, and numbers of concomitant medications is insignificant.

The problem is, that, if scores "zero to eight" are used as a linear covariate in a logistic model, then we assume that the risk of adverse-drug effect-admissions rises linearly, but this needs not to be so. If the relationship is a stepping function, like with categories, and, if we assume a linear relationship, then we are at risk of severely underestimating effects. In order to escape this risk, it is more appropriate to transform a quantitative estimator used as continuous variable into a categorical one. Using logistic regression in SPSS is convenient for the purpose, we need not manually transform the quantitative estimator. For the analysis we apply the usual commands: analyze. . . .regression. . . .binary logistic. . . .enter dependent variable. . . .enter independent variables. Then, open dialog box labelled categorical variables, select co-medication and transfer it into the box categorical variables, then click continue. Co-medication is now transformed into a categorical variable. Click OK.

The underneath Table is in the output, and gives the results. The number of co-medications has become a very significant predictor of the risk of admissions due to adverse drug effects with a p-value of 0.004. Obviously, the numbers of co-medications is an independent predictor of adverse-drug-effect-admissions, although not in a linear way but rather in a categorical way. This predictor remains statistically significant even after adjustment for age, gender, and presence co-morbidity.

Variables in the Equation

		B	S.E.	Wald	df	Sig.	Exp(B)
Step 1[a]	VAR00001	-,024	,004	32,859	1	,000	,976
	VAR00002	,080	,117	,470	1	,493	1,084
	VAR00010			22,241	8	,004	
	VAR00010(1)	18,900	40199,059	,000	1	1,000	1,615E8
	VAR00010(2)	19,490	40199,059	,000	1	1,000	2,914E8
	VAR00010(3)	18,923	40199,059	,000	1	1,000	1,653E8
	VAR00010(4)	19,342	40199,059	,000	1	1,000	2,514E8
	VAR00010(5)	18,820	40199,059	,000	1	1,000	1,491E8
	VAR00010(6)	19,122	40199,059	,000	1	1,000	2,017E8
	VAR00010(7)	17,932	40199,059	,000	1	1,000	6,133E7
	VAR00010(8)	-1,109	56845,749	,000	1	1,000	,330
	VAR00009	,109	,076	2,047	1	,152	1,115
	Constant	25,804	40199,060	,000	1	,999	1,609E11

a. Variable(s) entered on step 1: VAR00001, VAR00002, VAR00010, VAR00009.

The same data as those from the above table is given above, but now co-medication has been recoded from a continuous into a categorical variable with 9 categories (zero to 8 co-medications), (p-values < 0.10 are defined statistically significant).

9.3 Balanced-Iterative-Reducing-Hierarchy for Efficacy Analysis

Birch multidimensional clustering was able to identify not only clusters of young patients with few co-medications and older patients with many co-medications, but also a large outlier cluster of patients of all ages and “exceptionally-high-numbers-of-co-medications”. This supports, that the cluster of patients at all ages and with very many co-medications is an outlier to be interpreted as a dependent adverse effect.

Graphs like data plots and regression lines are convenient for visualizing outliers in therapeutic data patterns, and have been successfully used for that purpose for centuries. They are, however, arbitrary, and, with large data files, both data pattern and outlier recognition require a more sophisticated approach. Also, the number of outliers, generally, tends to rise linearly with the sample size. BIRCH is the abbreviation of "balanced iterative reducing and clustering using hierarchies", and is available in SPSS's module Classify, under "two-step cluster analysis". It is an unsupervised data mining methodology suitable for very large datasets, but can also be applied for small data. It is, currently, mainly used by econo- and sociometrists, and, like other machine learning methods, little used in therapeutic research. This is, probably, due to the traditional belief of clinicians in clinical trials where outliers are assumed to be equally balanced by the randomization process and are not further taken into account. In contrast, modern computer data files often involve large uncontrolled data files, and arbitrary methods like scatter plots do not adequately detect outliers in the data.

BIRCH clustering is able to detect previously unrecognized outlier data. Step by step analyses were performed for the convenience of investigators. This chapter was also written as a hand-hold presentation accessible to clinicians and a must read publication for those new to the method.

Example 1

The underneath table shows again the data of the above study of 50 mentally depressed patients. Age and depression severity scores (1 for mild and 10 for severest depression) are given in the first and second column. The cluster membership computed by two step BIRCH clustering is in column 3: two clusters were identified (indicated with 1 and 2) and one outlier cluster (indicated with −1)

Age	Depression score	Cluster membership
20,00	8,00	2
21,00	7,00	2
23,00	9,00	2
24,00	10,00	2
25,00	8,00	2
26,00	9,00	2
27,00	7,00	2
28,00	8,00	2
24,00	9,00	2
32,00	9,00	2
30,00	1,00	-1
40,00	2,00	-1
50,00	3,00	1
60,00	1,00	-1
70,00	2,00	1
76,00	3,00	1
65,00	2,00	1
54,00	3,00	1
54,00	4,00	1
49,00	3,00	1
30,00	4,00	2
25,00	5,00	2
24,00	4,00	2
27,00	5,00	2
35,00	6,00	2
45,00	5,00	1
45,00	6,00	2
67,00	7,00	1
80,00	6,00	1
80,00	5,00	1
40,00	1,00	-1
50,00	2,00	1
60,00	3,00	1
80,00	4,00	1
50,00	5,00	1
76,00	6,00	1
65,00	7,00	1
79,00	8,00	-1
57,00	3,00	1
46,00	4,00	1
54,00	5,00	1
74,00	6,00	1
65,00	7,00	1
57,00	9,00	-1
68,00	8,00	-1
67,00	7,00	1
65,00	6,00	1
64,00	5,00	1
74,00	4,00	1
75,00	3,00	1

Age and depression severity scores (1 for mild and 10 for severest depression) are given in the first and second column. Linear regression between the two variables gave some evidence for a weak negative correlation between the two with $p = 0.063$.

This would be compatible with the concept that younger are more at risk of high severity due to true depression, the older are so of low severity due to reactive depression. However, in case-reviews outlier forms of depression like insomnia groups have been noted, but no hints of such is given in the regression model. Even the 90% confidence intervals produced no more than a single case very close to the intervals boundary but otherwise no hint of outliers (figure below). An outlier analysis using two step BIRCH analysis was performed. SPSS statistical software was used for analysis.

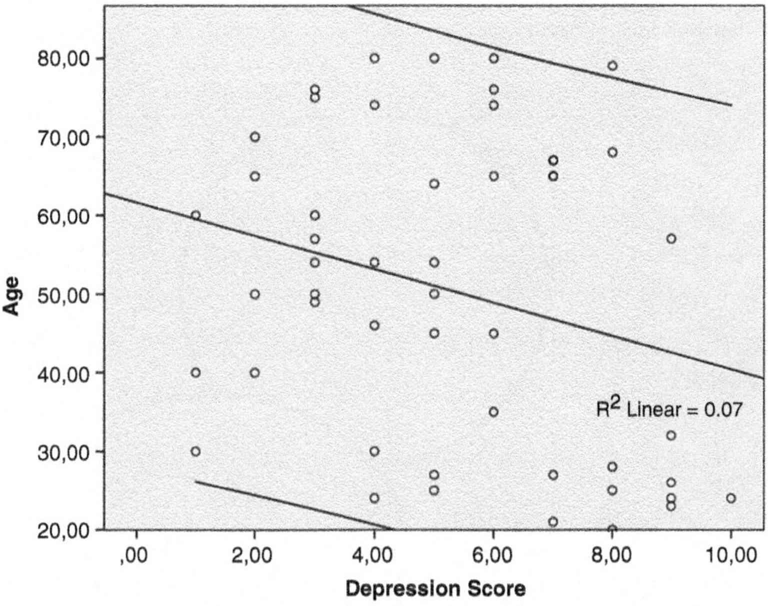

The SPSS data file is in extras.springer.com, and is entitled "birch1". Start by opening the data file in your computer mounted with SPSS statistical software.

Command Analyze....Classify....Two Step Cluster Analysis ....Continuous Variables: enter age and depression score....Distance Measure: mark Euclidean....Clustering Criterion: mark Schwarz's Bayesian Criterion....click Options: mark Use noise handling ....percentage: enter 25....Assumed Standardized: enter age and depression score....click Continue....click Output: Working Data File: mark Create cluster membership variable....click Continue....click OK.

When returning to the data file, it now shows the cluster membership of each case 1–50 (third column). Two clusters have been identified (indicated by 1 and 2) and one outlier cluster (indicated by −1). We will use SPSS again to draw a dotter graph of these results.

Command Analyze....Graphs....Legacy Dialogs: click Simple Scatter .... Define....Y-axis: enter Age....X-axis: enter Depression score....OK.

The underneath figure shows two clusters with oval and, because of the similarly sized scales, even approximately round patterns. They are also approximately similar in size but this needs not to be so. Also, 7 outlier data are shown. The results do very well match the patterns as clinically expected: two populations, one with younger and severely patients with true depression and one with older and milder depressed patients with only a reactive depression. The outliers consist of 7 patients of all ages not fitting in the formed clusters. They may suffer from insomnia or other rare forms of the depression syndrome.

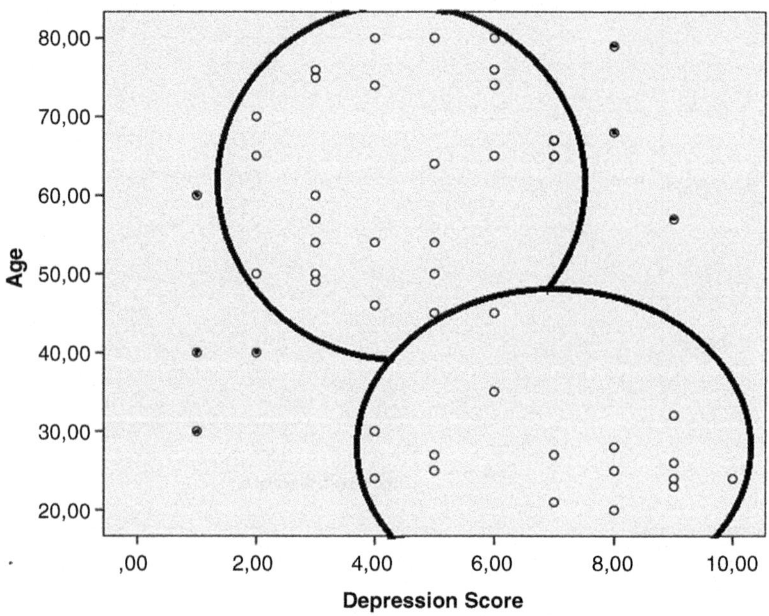

Thus, outlier detection using two step cluster analysis in SPSS identified two cluster and one outlier data set is. The lower cluster was compatible with younger patients suffering from true depression, the upper cluster with older patients suffering from reactive depression. The outliers on the left and on the right side were 4 younger patients with low depression scores, and 3 older patients with high depression scores, and did not fit in the clusters formerly established.

Example 2
In the above 2000 patient study of hospital admissions 576 possibly iatrogenic were identified by a team of specialists. The number of concomitant medications (co-medications) was not a significant predictor of hospital admission in the logistic regression of the data, but when transformed into a categorical factor it was. In order to find an explanation for this finding, a BIRCH two step cluster analysis of these data was performed in SPSS.

Open the data file, entitled "birch2", in your computer mounted with SPSS statistical software.

Command Analyze....Classify....Two Step Cluster Analysis ....Continuous Variables: enter age and co-medications....Distance Measure: mark Euclidean.... Clustering Criterion: mark Schwarz's Bayesian Criterion....click Options: mark Use noise handling ....percentage: enter 25....Assumed Standardized: enter age and co-medications....click Continue....click Plot: mark Cluster pie chart....click Continue....click Output: Statistics....mark Descriptives by cluster....mark Cluster frequencies....mark Information Criterion ....Working Data File: mark Create cluster membership variable....click Continue....click OK.

The underneath table shows that 15 different cluster models have been assessed by the two-step BIRCH procedure (including 1–15 clusters). The precision of the different models, as estimated by the overall uncertainties measured by Schwarz's Bayesian Criterion (BIC) is given. With the 3 or 4 cluster models the smallest BIC was observed, and, thus, the most precise model.

Auto-Clustering

Number of Clusters	Schwarz's Bayesian Criterion (BIC)	BIC Change[a]	Ratio of BIC Changes[b]	Ratio of Distance Measures[c]
1	293,899			
2	277,319	-16,580	1,000	1,513
3	185,362	-91,957	5,546	1,463
4	178,291	-7,071	,426	1,007
5	197,946	19,654	-1,185	1,141
6	216,403	18,457	-1,113	1,159
7	236,467	20,064	-1,210	1,099
8	251,072	14,606	-,881	1,629
9	272,582	21,509	-1,297	1,125
10	291,641	19,059	-1,150	1,015
11	301,090	9,449	-,570	1,000
12	308,019	6,929	-,418	1,058
13	321,943	13,924	-,840	1,197
14	339,382	17,439	-1,052	1,074
15	361,262	21,880	-1,320	1,225

a. The changes are from the previous number of clusters in the table.

b. The ratios of changes are relative to the change for the two cluster solution.

c. The ratios of distance measures are based on the current number of clusters against the previous number of clusters.

The table below also in the output sheets, gives description information of the 4 cluster model selected from the 15 models from the above table.

Centroids

		age		comed	
		Mean	Std. Deviation	Mean	Std. Deviation
Cluster	1	1928,9227	6,50936	2,5028	,50138
	2	1933,7171	6,01699	,6250	,48572
	3	1956,8551	6,16984	1,0725	,64895
	Outlier (-1)	1939,7644	20,15623	2,4138	1,75395
	Combined	1936,8090	14,91570	1,8090	1,34681

In the table below are frequency information of the 4 cluster model selected from the 15 models.

Cluster Distribution

		N	% of Combined	% of Total
Cluster	1	181	31,4%	9,1%
	2	152	26,4%	7,6%
	3	69	12,0%	3,5%
	Outlier (-1)	174	30,2%	8,7%
	Combined	576	100,0%	28,8%
Excluded Cases		1424		71,2%
Total		2000		100,0%

Thus, the above tables give the results of autoclustering of the two-step BIRCH procedure. It can be observed that 15 different models are assessed (including 1–15 clusters). Also is shown something about the precision of the different models, as estimated by the overall uncertainties (or standard errors) of the models (measured by Schwarz's Bayesian Criterion (BIC) = n ln (standard error)^2 + k ln n, where n = sample size, ln = natural logarithm, k = number of clusters). With the 3 or 4 cluster models the smallest BIC was observed, and, thus, the mostly precise model. The 3 or 4 cluster model, including an outlier cluster, would, therefore, be an adequate choice for further assessment of the data. Finally, description and frequency information of the 4 cluster model are given. The underneath figure in the output draws a pie chart of the size of the 3 clusters and the outlier cluster.

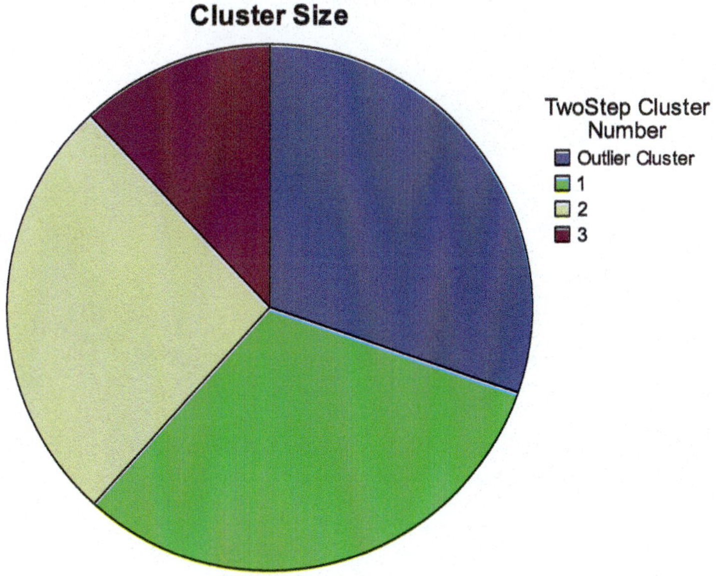

If we minimize the output pages, and return to the data file, we will observe, that SPSS has provided again the membership data. This file is too large to understand what is going on, and, therefore we will draw a three dimensional graph of this output.

Command Graphs....Legacy Dialogs....3 D Bar Charts....X-axis represents: click Groups of cases....Y- axis represents: click Groups of cases....click Define....Variable: enter co-medications....Bars represent: enter mean of values....X-Category axis: enter age....Y-Category axis: enter two step cluster number variable....click OK.

The figure below is shown in the output sheets. In front two clusters with younger patients and few co-medications are observed. In the third row is 1 cluster of elderly with considerably more co-medications. Then, at the back the patients are who do not fit in any of the clusters. They are of all ages, but their numbers of co-medications are generally very high. This finding is relevant, because it supports a deleterious effect of numbers of co-medications on the risk of iatrogenic admission.

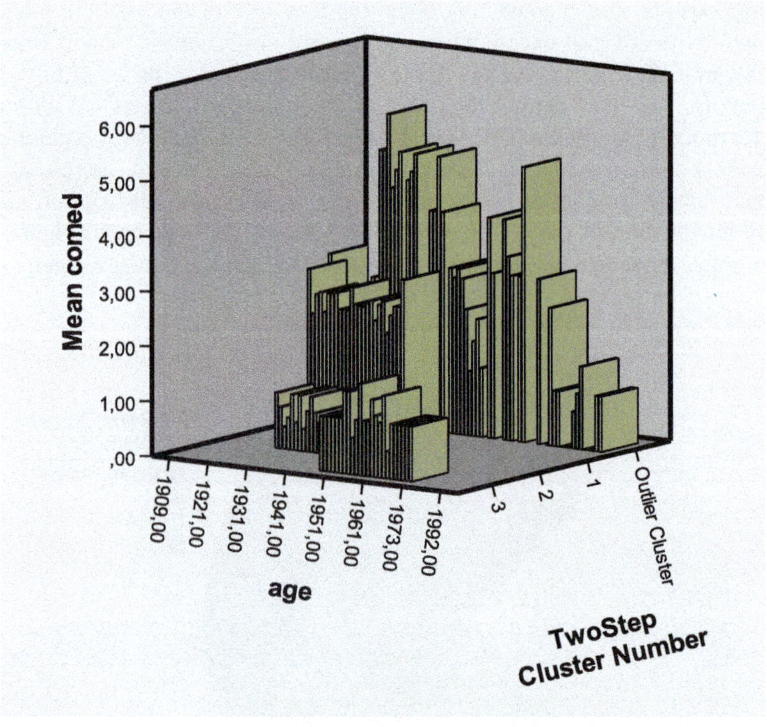

The above three-dimensional bar chart is selected from the 4 cluster model. Over 100 bars indicate mean numbers of co-medications in age classes of 1 year. In the clusters 2 and 3 the patients are young and have few co-medications, in the cluster 1 the patients are old and have many co-medications, in the outlier cluster all ages are present and exceptionally high numbers of co-medications are frequently observed.

The large outlier category consisted mainly of patients of all ages and extremely many co-medications. When returning to the Data View screen, we will observe that SPSS has created a novel variable entitled "TSC_5980" containing the patients' cluster memberships. The patients given the value −1 are the outliers.

With Scoring Wizard and the exported XML (eXtended Markup Language) file entitled "exportanomalydetection" we can now try and predict from age and number of co-medications (comed) of future patients the best fit cluster membership according to the computed XML model.

age	comed
1954,00	1,00
1938,00	7,00
1929,00	8,00
1967,00	1,00
1945,00	2,00
1936,00	3,00
1928,00	4,00

comed = number of co-medications

Enter the Above Data in a Novel Data File and Command

Utilities....click Scoring Wizard....click Browse....Open the appropriate folder with the XML file entitled "exportanomalydetection"....click on the latter and click Select....in Scoring Wizard double-click Next....mark Predicted Value ....click Finish.

age	comed	PredictedValue
1954,00	1,00	3,00
1938,00	7,00	−1,00
1929,00	8,00	−1,00
1967,00	1,00	3,00
1945,00	2,00	−1,00
1936,00	3,00	1,00
1928,00	4,00	−1,00

PredictedValue = predicted cluster membership

In the above novel data file SPSS has provided the new variable as requested. One patient is in cluster 1, two are in cluster 3, and 4 patients are in the outlier cluster.

An XML (eXtended Markup Language) file from a 2000 patient sample is, thus, capable of making predictions about cluster memberships and outlierships in future patients from the same target population.

9.4 Discussion

There is no rigorous mathematical definition for outliers of a dataset, unlike there is for, for example, p-values, r-values etc. Why then worry about the outliers after all? This is, because they can lead not only to serious misinterpretations of the data, but also to catastrophic consequences once the data are used for making predictions, like serious and, sometimes, even fatal adverse events from drug treatments.

The current chapter shows that traditional methods like regression analysis is often unable to demonstrate outliers, while outlier detection using BIRCH two step clustering is more successful to that aim. We should add that this clustering method points to remote points in the data and flags them as potential outliers. It does not confirm any other prior expectation about the nature or pattern of the outliers.

The outliers, generally, involve both extremely high and extremely low values. The approach is, obviously, explorative, but, as shown in the examples, it can produce interesting findings, and theories, although waiting for confirmation. Other forms of cluster analysis include hierarchical, k-means and density-based clustering. Although they can produce multiple clusters, they do not explicitly allow for an outlier option. Nonetheless, investigators are, of course, free to make interpretations about outlier clusters from the patterns as presented.

This chapter only addresses two-dimensional data (one x and one y-variable), but, similarly to multiple regression, BIRCH analysis can be used for analyzing multidimensional data, although the computations will rapidly become even more laborious and computer memory may rapidly fall short. In the future this kind of research will be increasingly performed through a network of computer systems rather than a single computer system let alone standalone computers. Also, multidimensional outliers may be harder to interpret, because they are associated with multiple factors.

This chapter addresses only outlier-assessment in data without outcome variables. If outcome variables are available, other methods can be used, particularly, the identification of data beyond the confidence limits of the outcome variables. Also some special methods are possible, then. For example, looking for the data that are closer to expectation than compatible with random distributions, and investigating the final digits of the data values.

Outlier recognition and removal is an adequate method for identifying and adjusting the adverse effect of the predictors on the outcome of a study with heterogeneous subgroups. In a study where age is studies to predict numbers of co-medications, and adjusted and removed outlier cluster is helpful to adjust the adverse effect of age on the numbers of co-medications

In this chapter traditional efficacy analysis, consistent of simple linear regressions, discretized continuous predictors, and multiple binary logistic regressions, was tested against the machine learning methodology called balanced iterative reducing hierarchy. Traditional efficacy analyses is often unable to demonstrate outliers, the BIRCH machine learning methodology was more successful for the purpose. Two data examples have been given. The machine learning analyses provided better sensitivity of testing, and were more informative.

9.5 References

To readers requesting more background, theoretical and mathematical information of computations given, several textbooks complementary to the current production and written by the same authors are available:

Statistics applied to clinical studies 5th edition, 2012,
Machine learning in medicine a complete overview, 2015,
SPSS for starters and 2nd levelers 2nd edition, 2015,
Clinical data analysis on a pocket calculator 2nd edition, 2016,
Understanding clinical data analysis from published research, 2016,
Modern meta-analysis, 2017,
Regression analysis in clinical research, 2018,
Modern Bayesian statistics in clinical research, 2018.
The Analysis of Safety Data of Drug Trials, an Update, 2019.

All of them have been edited by Springer Heidelberg Germany.

Chapter 10
Cluster-Analysis for Efficacy Analysis

Contents

Abstract In a parallel-group study of 50 depressed patients with different ages, the effect of ages on the levels of depression was tested, both traditionally, and with the help of machine learning.

Traditional efficacy analysis consisted of

discretization of continuous predictors,

simple linear regressions.

Machine learning efficacy analysis consisted of cluster-analysis methods.

The machine learning methods provided better sensitivity of testing, and were more informative.

Keywords Clinical trials · Traditional efficacy analysis · Machine learning efficacy analysis · Cluster-analysis methods

T. J. Cleophas, A. H. Zwinderman, *Efficacy Analysis in Clinical Trials an Update*,
https://doi.org/10.1007/978-3-030-19918-0_10

10.1 Introduction

Traditional efficacy analysis of parallel group studies of the effect of two age classes on an outcome can be analyzed with unpaired t-tests, or alternatively with a simple linear regression of the predictor age class on the outcome. A more informative approach to the analysis of such data is a cluster analysis. Various cluster models are available:

1. hierarchical cluster analysis
2. k-means cluster analysis
3. density-based cluster analysis.

Density-based clustering will be suitable, if small outlier groups between otherwise homogenous populations are expected. The other two will be more appropriate, if subgroups have a Gaussian-like pattern. In this chapter traditional efficacy analysis will be tested against the machine learning methodology called cluster analysis.

The traditional efficacy analysis will consist of discretized continuous predictors, and simple linear regressions.

10.2 Data Example

In a parallel group study of 50 depressed subjects of 2 age classes the effect of age class on level of depression was investigated. The same data have been applied in the previous chapter, but, instead of 40 years of age as cut-off for old and young, in this chapter 30 years of age was used. The age classes were, thus, classified according to patients of < 30 years and of > 30 years. The classification was consistent with the concept of severe endogenic depressions being more often diagnosed in the younger and less severe reactive depressions more often diagnosed in the older. SPSS statistical software was applied for classification of the age groups.

VAR 00001	00002	00003
age	depression score	patient number
20,00	8,00	1,00
21,00	7,00	2,00
23,00	9,00	3,00
24,00	10,00	4,00
25,00	8,00	5,00
26,00	9,00	6,00
27,00	7,00	7,00
28,00	8,00	8,00
24,00	9,00	9,00
32,00	9,00	10,00

The first 10 patients are above. The entire data file is entitled "hierkmeansdensity" and is in extras.springer.com. Start by opening the data file in your computer with SPSS statistical software installed (VAR = variable).

Command
Click Transform....Compute Variable....in Target Variable enter age....Numeric Expression: transfer VAR00001....add ">"....add "30"....click OK.

The Data View Screen now has a novel variable which is binary and is again entitled "age".

10.3 Traditional Efficacy Analysis

Traditional efficacy analysis consists of t-tests for continuous outcomes and chi-square tests for discrete outcomes. In Sect. 1.12, Chap. 1, the use of regression analyses for efficacy analyses is discussed, and in Sect. 1.13 the use of clinical trials for the assessment of causal health effects of factors other than medicines is discussed. For example, effects of interventions like angioplasties, surgeries, renal transplants etc. Many more factors can be tested in clinical trials, for example,

age factors
psychological factors
social factors
physical factors
economical factors,
and, any factor with a supposedly causal effect on health or sickness.

We will now perform a traditional simple linear regression with age class as predictor and depression score as scale measure outcome.

Command

Analyze. . . .Regression. . . .Linear. . . .Dependent: enter VAR00002. . . .Independent (s): enter age (age class). . . .click OK.

The underneath tables in the output show, that the "intervention" age class significantly predicts the outcome depression score (ANOVA = analysis of variance). The younger (< 30) have a significantly higher depression score than the older at p = 0.008.

Variables Entered/Removed[b]

Model	Variables Entered	Variables Removed	Method
1	age[a]	.	Enter

a. All requested variables entered.
b. Dependent Variable: VAR00002

Model Summary

Model	R	R Square	Adjusted R Square	Std. Error of the Estimate
1	,370[a]	,137	,119	2,32063

a. Predictors: (Constant), age

ANOVA[b]

Model		Sum of Squares	df	Mean Square	F	Sig.
1	Regression	41,124	1	41,124	7,636	,008[a]
	Residual	258,496	48	5,385		
	Total	299,620	49			

a. Predictors: (Constant), age
b. Dependent Variable: VAR00002

Coefficients[a]

Model		Unstandardized Coefficients		Standardized Coefficients	t	Sig.
		B	Std. Error	Beta		
1	(Constant)	6,714	,620		10,826	,000
	age	-2,020	,731	-,370	-2,763	,008

a. Dependent Variable: VAR00002

As an alternative, and, maybe, more informative approach to the analysis of these data cluster analyses can be performed as well.

10.4 Cluster-Analysis for Efficacy Analysis

Clusters are subgroups in a survey estimated by the distances between the values needed to connect the patients, otherwise called cases. It is an important methodology in explorative data mining. Three methods will be applied.

10.4.1 Hierarchical Cluster Analysis

SPSS 19.0 will be used for data analysis. Start by opening the data file.

Command

Analyze….Classify….Hierarchical Cluster Analysis….enter variables….Label Case by: case variable with the values 1-50….Plots: mark Dendrogram….Method ….Cluster Method: Between-group linkage….Measure: Squared Euclidean Distance….Save: click Single solution….Number of clusters: enter 3….Continue ….click OK.

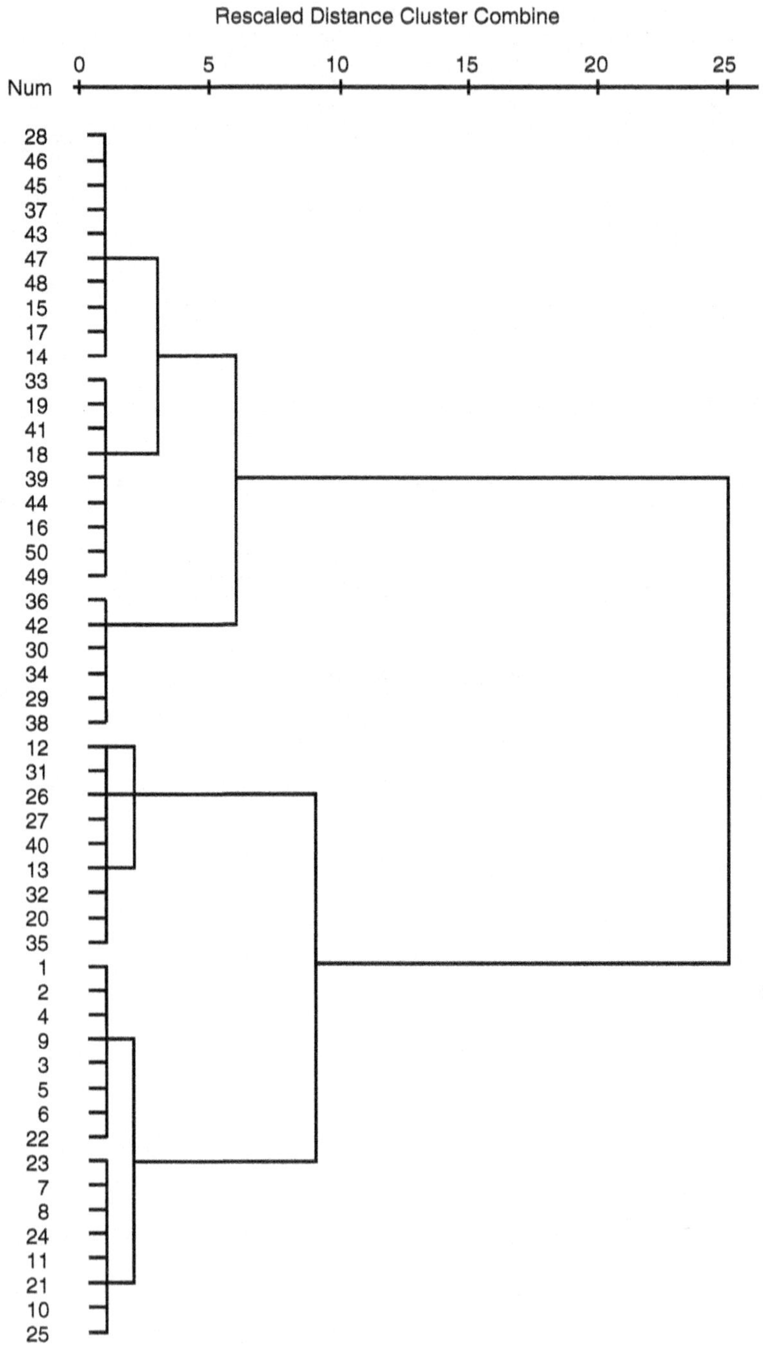
Rescaled Distance Cluster Combine
0
5
10
15
20
25
Num
28
46
45
37
43
47
48
15
17
14
33
19
41
18
39
44
16
50
49
36
42
30
34
29
38
12
31
26
27
40
13
32
20
35
1
2
4
9
3
5
6
22
23
7
8
24
11
21
10
25

In the output a dendrogram of the results is given. The actual distances between the cases are rescaled to fall into a range of 0–25 units (0 = minimal distance, 25 = maximal distance). The cases no. 1–11, 21–25 are clustered together in cluster 1, the cases 12, 13, 20, 26, 27, 31, 32, 35, 40 in cluster 2, both at a rescaled distance from 0 at approximately 3 units, the remainder of the cases is clustered at approximately 6 units. And so, as requested, three clusters have been indentified with cases more similar to one another than to the other clusters. When minimizing the output, the data file comes up and it now shows the cluster membership of each case. We will use SPSS again to draw a Dotter graph of the data.

Command

Analyze....Graphs....Legacy Dialogs: click Simple Scatter....Define....Y-axis: enter Depression Score....X-axis: enter Age....OK.

The graph (with age on the x-axis and severity score on the y-axis) produced by SPSS shows the cases. Using Microsoft's drawing commands we can encircle the clusters as identified. All of them are oval and even, approximately, round, because variables have similar scales, but they are different in size.

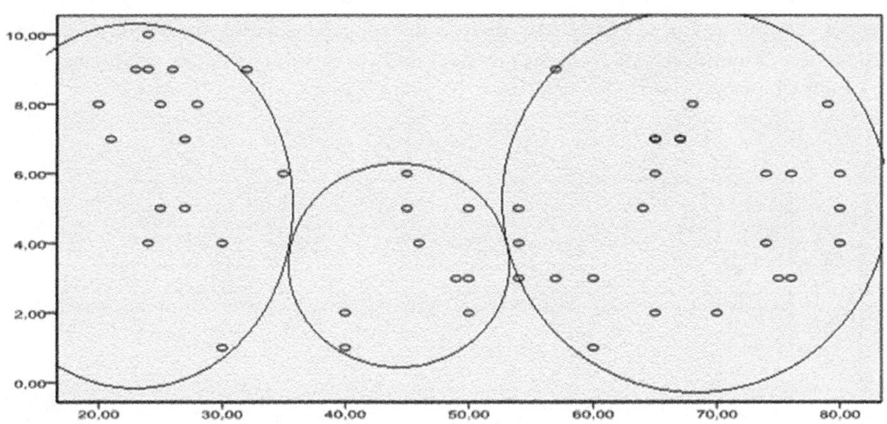

10.4.2 K-Means Cluster Analysis

Command

Analyze....Classify....K-means Cluster Analysis....Variables: enter Age and Depression score....Label Cases by: patient number as a string variable....Number of clusters: 3 (in our example chosen for comparison with the above method).... click Method: mark Iterate....click Iterate: Maximal Iterations: mark 10.... Convergence criterion: mark 0....click Continue....click Save: mark Cluster Membership....click Continue....click Options: mark Initiate cluster centers.... mark ANOVA table....mark Cluster information for each case....click Continue ....click OK.

The output shows that the three clusters identified by the k-means cluster model were significantly different from one another both by testing the y-axis (depression score) and the x-axis variable (age). When minimizing the output sheets, the data file comes up and shows the cluster membership of the three clusters.

ANOVA

	Cluster		Error		F	Sig.
	Mean Square	df	Mean Square	df		
Age	8712,723	2	31,082	47	280,310	,000
Depression Score	39,102	2	4,593	47	8,513	,001

We will use SPSS again to draw a Dotter graph of the data.

Command

Analyze....Graphs....Legacy Dialogs: click Simple Scatter....Define....Y-axis: enter Depression Score....X-axis: enter Age....click OK.

The graph (with age on the x-axis and severity score on the y-axis) produced by SPSS shows the cases. Using Microsoft's drawing commands we can encircle the clusters as identified. All of them are oval and even approximately round because variables have similar scales, and they are approximately equal in size.

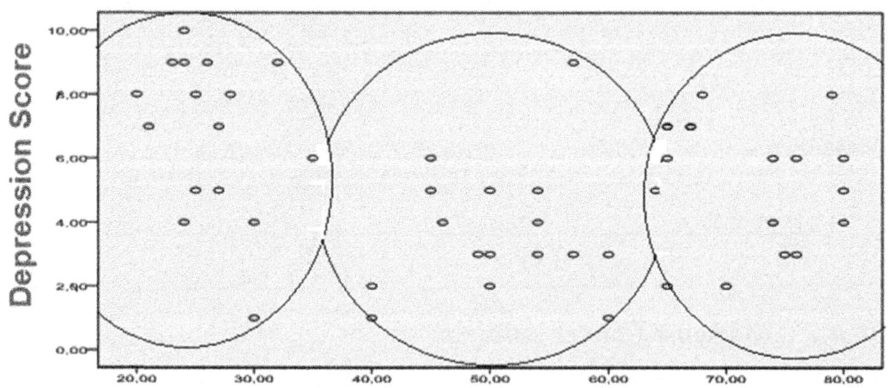

Clusters are estimated by the distances between the values needed to connect the cases. It is an important methodology in explorative data mining. Hierarchical clustering is adequate, if subgroups are expected to be different in size, k-means clustering if approximately similar in size. Density-based clustering is more appropriate, if small outlier groups between otherwise homogenous populations are expected.

10.4.3 Density-Based Cluster Analysis

The DBSCAN method was used (density based spatial clustering of application with noise). As this method is not available in SPSS, an interactive JAVA Applet freely available at the Internet was used [Data Clustering Applets. http://webdocs.cs.ualberts.ca/~yaling/Cluster/applet]. The DBSCAN connects points that satisfy a density criterion given by a minimum number of patients within a defined radius (radius = Eps; minimum number = Min pts).

Command

User Define....Choose data set: remove values given....enter you own x and y values....Choose algorithm: select DBSCAN....Eps: mark 25....Min pts: mark 3....Start....Show.

Three cluster memberships are again shown. We will use SPSS 19.0 again to draw a Dotter graph of the data.

Command

Analyze....Graphs....Legacy Dialogs: click Simple Scatter....Define....Y-axis: enter Depression Score....X-axis: enter Age....click OK.

The graph (with age on the x-axis and severity score on the y-axis) shows the cases. Using Microsoft's drawing commands we can encircle the clusters as identified. Two very small ones, one large one. All of the clusters identified are non-circular and, are, obviously, based on differences in patient-density.

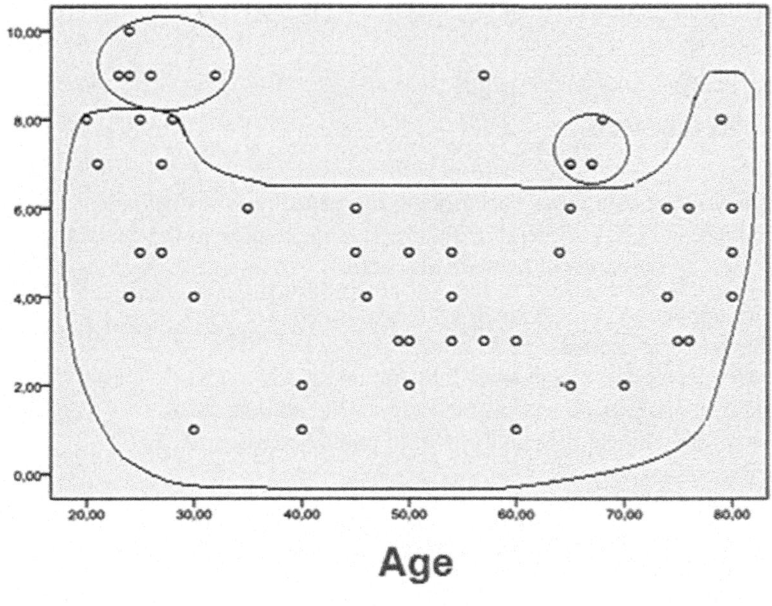

Clusters are estimated by the distances between the values needed to connect the cases. It is an important methodology in explorative data mining. Density-based clustering is suitable, if small outlier groups between otherwise homogeneous populations are expected. Hierarchical and k-means clustering are more appropriate, if subgroups have Gaussian-like patterns.

10.5 Discussion

Traditional efficacy analysis of a parallel group studies of an effect on an outcome can be analyzed with unpaired t-tests, or alternatively with a simple linear regression of the predictor age class on the outcome. An alternative, and maybe sometimes more informative approach to the analysis of such data is a cluster analysis. Various cluster models are available:

1. hierarchical cluster analysis
2. k-means cluster analysis
3. density-based cluster analysis.

Density-based clustering are suitable, if small outlier groups between otherwise homogenous populations are expected. The other two are more appropriate if subgroups have a Gaussian-like pattern. The example of this chapter shows, that cluster models provide relevant new patterns in parallel group data. In this chapter traditional efficacy analysis, consistent of discretized continuous predictors and simple linear regressions were tested against the machine learning methodology called cluster analysis. The machine learning analyses provided better sensitivity of testing, and were more informative.

10.6 References

To readers requesting more background, theoretical and mathematical information of computations given, several textbooks complementary to the current production and written by the same authors are available:

Statistics applied to clinical studies 5th edition, 2012,
Machine learning in medicine a complete overview, 2015,
SPSS for starters and 2nd levelers 2nd edition, 2015,
Clinical data analysis on a pocket calculator 2nd edition, 2016,
Understanding clinical data analysis from published research, 2016,
Modern meta-analysis, 2017,
Regression analysis in clinical research, 2018,
Modern Bayesian statistics in clinical research, 2018.
The Analysis of Safety Data of Drug Trials, an Update, 2019.

All of them have been edited by Springer Heidelberg Germany.

Chapter 11
Multidimensional-Scaling for Efficacy Analysis

Contents

Abstract In 42 patients the effects of the random administrations of 15 different pain-killers on preference scoring was tested, both traditionally, and with the help of machine learning.

Traditional efficacy analysis consisted of

paired t-tests,
confidence intervals,
equivalence testing.

Machine learning efficacy analysis consisted of multidimensional-scaling methods.

The machine learning methods provided better sensitivity of testing, and were more informative.

Keywords Clinical trials · Traditional efficacy analysis · Machine learning efficacy analysis · Multidimensional-scaling methods

11.1 Introduction

To individual patients, objective criteria of drug efficacy, like pharmaco-dynamic-kinetic and safety measures may not mean too much, and patients' personal opinions are important too. Traditionally paired t-tests can used to test the significance of difference between mean preference scores for one drug versus the other

T. J. Cleophas, A. H. Zwinderman, *Efficacy Analysis in Clinical Trials an Update*,
https://doi.org/10.1007/978-3-030-19918-0_11

followed by equivalence testing of mean preference differences in the data. But the overall result may be pretty inconclusive, and multidimensional scaling may be better sensitive for the purpose. In this chapter a traditional efficacy analysis will be tested against the machine learning methodology called multidimensional scaling. The traditional efficacy analysis will consist of paired t-tests, confidence intervals, and equivalence testing.

11.2 Traditional Efficacy Analysis

Traditional efficacy analysis consists of t-tests for continuous outcomes and chi-square tests for discrete outcomes. In Sect. 1.12, Chap. 1, the use of regression analyses for efficacy analyses is discussed, and in Sect. 1.13 the use of clinical trials for the assessment of causal health effects of factors other than medicines is discussed. For example, effects of interventions like angioplasties, surgeries, renal transplants etc. Many more factors can be tested in clinical trials, for example,

age factors
psychological factors
social factors
physical factors
economical factors,
and, any factor with a supposedly causal effect on health or sickness.

In a prospective study of preference ranking of the 15 pain killers, 42 patients were tested 15 times in a randomized crossover setting. Part of the data file is underneath.

Var 1	2	3	4	5	6	7	8	9	10	11	12	13	14	15
12	13	7	4	5	2	8	10	11	14	3	1	6	9	15
14	11	6	3	10	4	15	8	9	12	7	1	5	2	13
13	10	12	14	3	2	9	8	7	11	1	6	4	5	15
7	14	11	3	6	8	12	10	9	15	4	1	2	5	13
14	9	6	15	13	2	11	8	7	10	12	1	3	4	5
9	11	15	4	7	6	14	10	8	12	5	2	3	1	13
9	14	5	6	8	4	13	11	12	15	7	2	1	3	10
15	10	12	6	8	2	13	9	7	11	3	1	5	4	14
13	12	2	4	5	8	10	11	3	15	7	9	6	1	14
15	13	10	7	6	4	9	11	12	14	5	2	8	1	3
9	2	4	13	8	5	1	10	6	7	11	15	14	12	3

Var 1–15 preference scores (1 = most prefered, 15 = least prefered)

Only the first 11 patients are given. The entire data file is entitled "prefscal" and is in extras.springer.com.

To 42 patients 15 different pain-killers are administered, and the patients are requested to rank them in order of preference from 1 "most prefered" to 15 "least prefered".

First we will make a plot of mean preference scores from the above data. Then, paired samples t-tests will be performed of all pain-killers versus one another. According to the protocol an equivalence analysis was performed of mean preference differences and their 95% confidence intervals (CIs). The a priori defined D-boundaries of equivalence were between −3 and + 3 score units. Non- equivalence was demonstrated of the differences between mean pain-killer scores if the 95% confidence intervals were < −3 or > +3 score units. The analysis was done in a computer with SPSS statistical software installed. Start by opening the data file.

Command

Graphs....Error Bars....click Simple....mark Sums of separate variables....click Define....Error Bars: enter pain-killer 1 to 15....Bars Represent...mark Confidence interval for mean....level %: enter 95....click OK.

The underneath graph was in the output sheets.

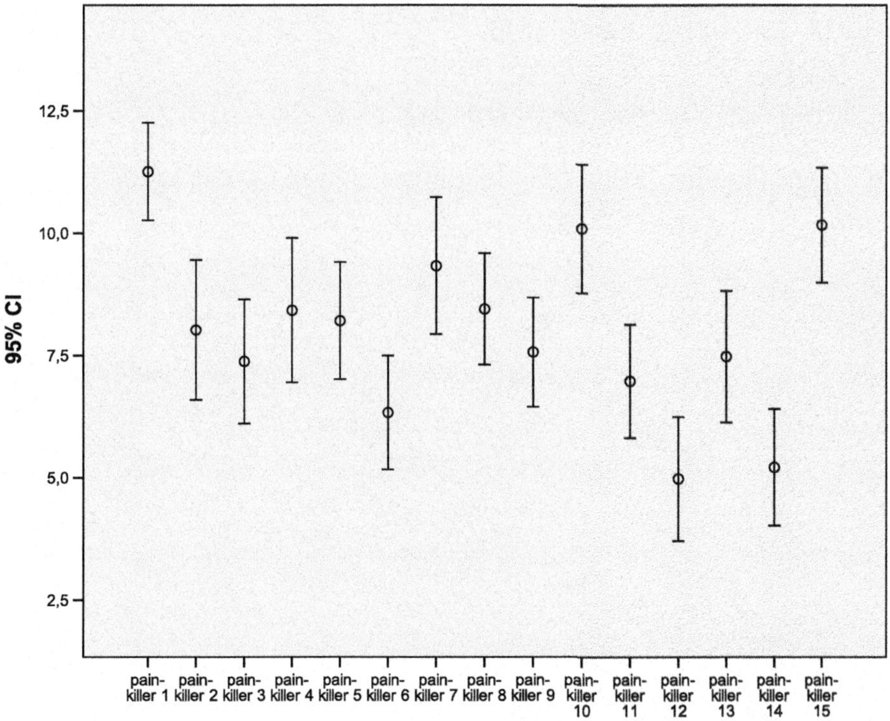

The pain-killers 1, 10, and 15 have the highest scores, the pain-killers 12 and 14 the lowest. We wish to know, whether and when the confidence intervals of the differences between two pain-killers are larger or smaller than the D-boundaries of equivalence, as set a priori between −3 and +3 score units.

Command

Analyze....Compare Means....Paired-Samples T Test....Paired Variables: enter

	Variable 1	Variable 2
Pair 1	pain-killer 1	pain-killer 2
Pair 2	pain-killer 1	pain-killer 3
Pair 3	pain-killer 1	pain-killer 4
Pair 4	pain-killer 1	pain-killer 5
Pair 5	pain-killer 1	pain-killer 6
Pair 6	pain-killer 1	pain-killer 7
Pair 7	pain-killer 1	pain-killer 8
Pair 8	pain-killer 1	pain-killer 9
Pair 9	pain-killer 1	pain-killer 10
Pair 10	pain-killer 1	pain-killer 11
Pair 11	pain-killer 1	pain-killer 12
Pair 12	pain-killer 1	pain-killer 13
Pair 13	pain-killer 1	pain-killer 14
Pair 14	pain-killer 1	pain-killer 15

click OK.

In the output sheets the underneath table is given.

Paired Samples Test

		Paired Differences					t	df	Sig. (2-tailed)
					95% Confidence Interval of the Difference				
		Mean	Std. Deviation	Std. Error Mean	Lower	Upper			
Pair 1	pain-killer 1 - pain-killer 2	3,238	5,450	,841	1,540	4,936	3,851	41	,000
Pair 2	pain-killer 1 - pain-killer 3	3,881	5,451	,841	2,182	5,580	4,614	41	,000
Pair 3	pain-killer 1 - pain-killer 4	2,833	5,360	,827	1,163	4,504	3,426	41	,001
Pair 4	pain-killer 1 - pain-killer 5	3,048	5,785	,893	1,245	4,850	3,414	41	,001
Pair 5	pain-killer 1 - pain-killer 6	4,929	5,321	,821	3,270	6,587	6,003	41	,000
Pair 6	pain-killer 1 - pain-killer 7	1,929	5,488	,847	,218	3,639	2,277	41	,028
Pair 7	pain-killer 1 - pain-killer 8	2,810	4,479	,691	1,414	4,205	4,065	41	,000
Pair 8	pain-killer 1 - pain-killer 9	3,690	4,688	,723	2,230	5,151	5,102	41	,000
Pair 9	pain-killer 1 - pain-killer 10	1,167	5,273	,814	-,476	2,810	1,434	41	,159
Pair 10	pain-killer 1 - pain-killer 11	4,286	5,009	,773	2,725	5,847	5,545	41	,000
Pair 11	pain-killer 1 - pain-killer 12	6,286	5,366	,828	4,614	7,958	7,591	41	,000
Pair 12	pain-killer 1 - pain-killer 13	3,786	5,426	,837	2,095	5,477	4,522	41	,000
Pair 13	pain-killer 1 - pain-killer 14	6,048	5,889	,909	4,212	7,883	6,655	41	,000
Pair 14	pain-killer 1 - pain-killer 15	1,095	5,254	,811	-,542	2,732	1,351	41	,184

Obviously, many one by one comparisons were statistically significant at $p < 0.05$, but equivalence, as measured with score units > 3 or < −3, could only be rejected rarely.

Pain-killer 1 versus 6 produced a 95% CI of 6.587 - 3.270 = 3.317
Pain-killer 1 versus 13 ....= 3.382
Pain-killer 1 versus 15 ....= 3.671.

Next, paired t-tests of all of the remaining one by one paired comparisons were performed giving similar commands. The output is below.

pain-killer 2 versus 3-15

Paired Samples Test

		Paired Differences					t	df	Sig. (2-tailed)
					95% Confidence Interval of the Difference				
		Mean	Std. Deviation	Std. Error Mean	Lower	Upper			
Pair 1	pain-killer 2 - pain-killer 3	,643	5,742	,886	-1,146	2,432	,726	41	,472
Pair 2	pain-killer 2 - pain-killer 4	-,405	7,967	1,229	-2,887	2,078	-,329	41	,744
Pair 3	pain-killer 2 - pain-killer 5	-,190	6,352	,980	-2,170	1,789	-,194	41	,847
Pair 4	pain-killer 2 - pain-killer 6	1,690	6,838	1,055	-,440	3,821	1,602	41	,117
Pair 5	pain-killer 2 - pain-killer 7	-1,310	3,632	,560	-2,441	-,178	-2,336	41	,024
Pair 6	pain-killer 2 - pain-killer 8	-,429	5,042	,778	-2,000	1,143	-,551	41	,585
Pair 7	pain-killer 2 - pain-killer 9	,452	4,549	,702	-,965	1,870	,644	41	,523
Pair 8	pain-killer 2 - pain-killer 10	-2,071	3,990	,616	-3,315	-,828	-3,364	41	,002
Pair 9	pain-killer 2 - pain-killer 11	1,048	7,574	1,169	-1,313	3,408	,896	41	,375
Pair 10	pain-killer 2 - pain-killer 12	3,048	7,651	1,181	,663	5,432	2,582	41	,014
Pair 11	pain-killer 2 - pain-killer 13	,548	7,775	1,200	-1,875	2,970	,456	41	,650
Pair 12	pain-killer 2 - pain-killer 14	2,810	7,706	1,189	,408	5,211	2,363	41	,023
Pair 13	pain-killer 2 - pain-killer 15	-2,143	5,779	,892	-3,944	-,342	-2,403	41	,021

pain-killer 3 versus 4-15

Paired Samples Test

		Paired Differences					t	df	Sig. (2-tailed)
					95% Confidence Interval of the Difference				
		Mean	Std. Deviation	Std. Error Mean	Lower	Upper			
Pair 1	pain-killer 3 - pain-killer 4	-1,048	7,418	1,145	-3,359	1,264	-,915	41	,365
Pair 2	pain-killer 3 - pain-killer 5	-,833	5,137	,793	-2,434	,767	-1,051	41	,299
Pair 3	pain-killer 3 - pain-killer 6	1,048	4,854	,749	-,465	2,560	1,399	41	,169
Pair 4	pain-killer 3 - pain-killer 7	-1,952	5,530	,853	-3,676	-,229	-2,288	41	,027
Pair 5	pain-killer 3 - pain-killer 8	-1,071	6,326	,976	-3,043	,900	-1,098	41	,279
Pair 6	pain-killer 3 - pain-killer 9	-,190	5,807	,896	-2,000	1,619	-,213	41	,833
Pair 7	pain-killer 3 - pain-killer 10	-2,714	5,597	,864	-4,459	-,970	-3,143	41	,003
Pair 8	pain-killer 3 - pain-killer 11	,405	5,972	,921	-1,456	2,266	,439	41	,663
Pair 9	pain-killer 3 - pain-killer 12	2,405	6,928	1,069	,246	4,564	2,249	41	,030
Pair 10	pain-killer 3 - pain-killer 13	-,095	6,942	1,071	-2,258	2,068	-,089	41	,930
Pair 11	pain-killer 3 - pain-killer 14	2,167	5,486	,846	,457	3,876	2,560	41	,014
Pair 12	pain-killer 3 - pain-killer 15	-2,786	5,082	,784	-4,370	-1,202	-3,552	41	,001

pain-killer 4 versus 5-15

Paired Samples Test

		Paired Differences					t	df	Sig. (2-tailed)
					95% Confidence Interval of the Difference				
		Mean	Std. Deviation	Std. Error Mean	Lower	Upper			
Pair 1	pain-killer 4 - pain-killer 5	,214	6,535	1,008	-1,822	2,251	,212	41	,833
Pair 2	pain-killer 4 - pain-killer 6	2,095	6,385	,985	,105	4,085	2,127	41	,040
Pair 3	pain-killer 4 - pain-killer 7	-,905	8,165	1,260	-3,449	1,640	-,718	41	,477
Pair 4	pain-killer 4 - pain-killer 8	-,024	6,583	1,016	-2,075	2,028	-,023	41	,981
Pair 5	pain-killer 4 - pain-killer 9	,857	6,517	1,006	-1,174	2,888	,852	41	,399
Pair 6	pain-killer 4 - pain-killer 10	-1,667	7,404	1,142	-3,974	,640	-1,459	41	,152
Pair 7	pain-killer 4 - pain-killer 11	1,452	4,490	,693	,053	2,851	2,097	41	,042
Pair 8	pain-killer 4 - pain-killer 12	3,452	4,290	,662	2,116	4,789	5,216	41	,000
Pair 9	pain-killer 4 - pain-killer 13	,952	4,596	,709	-,480	2,384	1,343	41	,187
Pair 10	pain-killer 4 - pain-killer 15	-1,738	7,302	1,127	-4,014	,537	-1,543	41	,131
Pair 11	pain-killer 4 - pain-killer 14	3,214	5,367	,828	1,542	4,887	3,881	41	,000

pain-killer 5 versus 6-15

Paired Samples Test

		Paired Differences					t	df	Sig. (2-tailed)
					95% Confidence Interval of the Difference				
		Mean	Std. Deviation	Std. Error Mean	Lower	Upper			
Pair 1	pain-killer 5 - pain-killer 6	1,881	5,283	,815	,235	3,527	2,307	41	,026
Pair 2	pain-killer 5 - pain-killer 7	-1,119	6,379	,984	-3,107	,869	-1,137	41	,262
Pair 3	pain-killer 5 - pain-killer 8	-,238	5,767	,890	-2,035	1,559	-,268	41	,790
Pair 4	pain-killer 5 - pain-killer 9	,643	5,021	,775	-,922	2,208	,830	41	,411
Pair 5	pain-killer 5 - pain-killer 10	-1,881	6,398	,987	-3,875	,113	-1,905	41	,064
Pair 6	pain-killer 5 - pain-killer 11	1,238	4,611	,711	-,199	2,675	1,740	41	,089
Pair 7	pain-killer 5 - pain-killer 12	3,238	6,393	,986	1,246	5,230	3,283	41	,002
Pair 8	pain-killer 5 - pain-killer 13	,738	5,902	,911	-1,101	2,577	,810	41	,422
Pair 9	pain-killer 5 - pain-killer 14	3,000	5,089	,785	1,414	4,586	3,820	41	,000
Pair 10	pain-killer 5 - pain-killer 15	-1,952	5,314	,820	-3,608	-,296	-2,381	41	,022

pain-killer 6 versus 7-15

Paired Samples Test

		Paired Differences					t	df	Sig. (2-tailed)
		Mean	Std. Deviation	Std. Error Mean	95% Confidence Interval of the Difference Lower	Upper			
Pair 1	pain-killer 6 - pain-killer 7	-3,000	6,607	1,020	-5,059	-,941	-2,942	41	,005
Pair 2	pain-killer 6 - pain-killer 8	-2,119	6,106	,942	-4,022	-,216	-2,249	41	,030
Pair 3	pain-killer 6 - pain-killer 9	-1,238	6,258	,966	-3,188	,712	-1,282	41	,207
Pair 4	pain-killer 6 - pain-killer 10	-3,762	6,324	,976	-5,733	-1,791	-3,855	41	,000
Pair 5	pain-killer 6 - pain-killer 11	-,643	5,060	,781	-2,220	,934	-,823	41	,415
Pair 6	pain-killer 6 - pain-killer 12	1,357	5,136	,793	-,243	2,958	1,712	41	,094
Pair 7	pain-killer 6 - pain-killer 13	-1,143	5,916	,913	-2,987	,701	-1,252	41	,218
Pair 8	pain-killer 6 - pain-killer 14	1,119	4,329	,668	-,230	2,468	1,675	41	,102
Pair 9	pain-killer 6 - pain-killer 15	-3,833	4,137	,638	-5,123	-2,544	-6,004	41	,000

pain-killer 7 versus 8-15

Paired Samples Test

		Paired Differences					t	df	Sig. (2-tailed)
		Mean	Std. Deviation	Std. Error Mean	95% Confidence Interval of the Difference Lower	Upper			
Pair 1	pain-killer 7 - pain-killer 8	,881	5,338	,824	-,783	2,544	1,069	41	,291
Pair 2	pain-killer 7 - pain-killer 9	1,762	5,364	,828	,090	3,433	2,129	41	,039
Pair 3	pain-killer 7 - pain-killer 10	-,762	4,438	,685	-2,145	,621	-1,113	41	,272
Pair 4	pain-killer 7 - pain-killer 11	2,357	7,005	1,081	,174	4,540	2,181	41	,035
Pair 5	pain-killer 7 - pain-killer 12	4,357	7,440	1,148	2,039	6,676	3,795	41	,000
Pair 6	pain-killer 7 - pain-killer 13	1,857	7,537	1,163	-,492	4,206	1,597	41	,118
Pair 7	pain-killer 7 - pain-killer 14	4,119	7,362	1,136	1,825	6,413	3,626	41	,001
Pair 8	pain-killer 7 - pain-killer 15	-,833	5,282	,815	-2,479	,813	-1,022	41	,313

pain-killer 8 versus 9-15

Paired Samples Test

		Paired Differences					t	df	Sig. (2-tailed)
					95% Confidence Interval of the Difference				
		Mean	Std. Deviation	Std. Error Mean	Lower	Upper			
Pair 1	pain-killer 8 - pain-killer 9	,881	3,877	,598	-,327	2,089	1,472	41	,149
Pair 2	pain-killer 8 - pain-killer 10	-1,643	5,031	,776	-3,211	-,075	-2,116	41	,040
Pair 3	pain-killer 8 - pain-killer 11	1,476	5,985	,923	-,389	3,341	1,599	41	,118
Pair 4	pain-killer 8 - pain-killer 12	3,476	5,654	,872	1,714	5,238	3,985	41	,000
Pair 5	pain-killer 8 - pain-killer 13	,976	6,079	,938	-,918	2,870	1,041	41	,304
Pair 6	pain-killer 8 - pain-killer 14	3,238	6,032	,931	1,358	5,118	3,479	41	,001
Pair 7	pain-killer 8 - pain-killer 15	-1,714	5,580	,861	-3,453	,025	-1,991	41	,053

pain-killer 9 versus 10-15

Paired Samples Test

		Paired Differences					t	df	Sig. (2-tailed)
					95% Confidence Interval of the Difference				
		Mean	Std. Deviation	Std. Error Mean	Lower	Upper			
Pair 1	pain-killer 9 - pain-killer 10	-2,524	5,452	,841	-4,223	-,825	-3,000	41	,005
Pair 2	pain-killer 9 - pain-killer 11	,595	6,065	,936	-1,295	2,485	,636	41	,528
Pair 3	pain-killer 9 - pain-killer 12	2,595	6,125	,945	,687	4,504	2,746	41	,009
Pair 4	pain-killer 9 - pain-killer 13	,095	5,971	,921	-1,765	1,956	,103	41	,918
Pair 5	pain-killer 9 - pain-killer 14	2,357	5,930	,915	,509	4,205	2,576	41	,014
Pair 6	pain-killer 9 - pain-killer 15	-2,595	5,575	,860	-4,332	-,858	-3,017	41	,004

pain-killer 10 versus 11-15

Paired Samples Test

		Paired Differences					t	df	Sig. (2-tailed)
					95% Confidence Interval of the Difference				
		Mean	Std. Deviation	Std. Error Mean	Lower	Upper			
Pair 1	pain-killer 10 - pain-killer 11	3,119	6,833	1,054	,990	5,248	2,958	41	,005
Pair 2	pain-killer 10 - pain-killer 12	5,119	6,689	1,032	3,035	7,203	4,960	41	,000
Pair 3	pain-killer 10 - pain-killer 13	2,619	6,925	1,068	,461	4,777	2,451	41	,019
Pair 4	pain-killer 10 - pain-killer 14	4,881	7,092	1,094	2,671	7,091	4,460	41	,000
Pair 5	pain-killer 10 - pain-killer 15	-,071	5,858	,904	-1,897	1,754	-,079	41	,937

pain-killer 11 versus 12-15

Paired Samples Test

		Paired Differences					t	df	Sig. (2-tailed)
					95% Confidence Interval of the Difference				
		Mean	Std. Deviation	Std. Error Mean	Lower	Upper			
Pair 1	pain-killer 11 - pain-killer 12	2,000	4,722	,729	,529	3,471	2,745	41	,009
Pair 2	pain-killer 11 - pain-killer 13	-,500	4,397	,678	-1,870	,870	-,737	41	,465
Pair 3	pain-killer 11 - pain-killer 14	1,762	4,189	,646	,456	3,067	2,726	41	,009
Pair 4	pain-killer 11 - pain-killer 15	-3,190	6,021	,929	-5,067	-1,314	-3,434	41	,001

pain-killer 12 versus 13-15

Paired Samples Test

		Paired Differences					t	df	Sig. (2-tailed)
		Mean	Std. Deviation	Std. Error Mean	95% Confidence Interval of the Difference Lower	Upper			
Pair 1	pain-killer 12 - pain-killer 13	-2,500	4,759	,734	-3,983	-1,017	-3,405	41	,001
Pair 2	pain-killer 12 - pain-killer 14	-,238	4,107	,634	-1,518	1,042	-,376	41	,709
Pair 3	pain-killer 12 - pain-killer 15	-5,190	6,062	,935	-7,079	-3,302	-5,549	41	,000

pain-killer 13 versus 14-15

Paired Samples Test

		Paired Differences					t	df	Sig. (2-tailed)
		Mean	Std. Deviation	Std. Error Mean	95% Confidence Interval of the Difference Lower	Upper			
Pair 1	pain-killer 13 - pain-killer 14	2,262	5,166	,797	,652	3,872	2,838	41	,007
Pair 2	pain-killer 13 - pain-killer 15	-2,690	6,773	1,045	-4,801	-,580	-2,574	41	,014

pain-killer 14 versus 15

Paired Samples Test

		Paired Differences					t	df	Sig. (2-tailed)
		Mean	Std. Deviation	Std. Error Mean	95% Confidence Interval of the Difference Lower	Upper			
Pair 1	pain-killer 14 - pain-killer 15	-4,952	5,046	,779	-6,525	-3,380	-6,361	41	,000

With D-boundaries from −3 to +3 units, non-equivalence would have been demonstrated, if the 95% confidence interval of the results were entirely < -3 or $> +3$. Again, obviously non-equivalence was demonstrated only rarely.

Namely:

difference between	pain-killer 1 and 6	1 is prefered.
	pain-killer 1 and 12	1 is prefered
	pain-killer 1 and 14	1 is prefered
	pain-killer 10 and 12	10 is prefered
	pain-killer 12 and 15	15 is prefered
	pain-killer 14 and 15	15 is prefered.

Obviously, the pain-killers 1, 10, and 15 have better scores than the rest compared to pain-killers 6, 12, and 14. However, the scores 1, 10, 15 are not better than all of the other scores, and, so, this traditional equivalence testing procedure leaves us with a pretty inconclusive overall result.

11.3 Multidimensional Scaling for Efficacy Analysis

Multidimensional scaling consists of proximity and preference scaling and is available in SPSS statistical software. We wish to assess whether proximity and preference scores of pain-killers as judged by patients can be used for obtaining insight in the real patients' priorities. For the purpose individual proximities or preferences are modeled in two-dimensional planes using the Pythagorian, otherwise called Euclidean equation with distances or proximities given by

$$\sqrt{\left[(x_i - x_j)^2 + \left(y_i - y_j\right)^2\right]}.$$

11.3.1 Proximity Scaling

An example is given.

The variables (Var 1–14) are one by one distance scores of the 14 pain-killers, they are the means of 20 patients (scale 0–10). The data file is given below, and also for convenience in extras.springer.com, entitled "proxscal".

Var	Var 1	Var 2	Var 3	Var 4	Var 5	Var 6	Var 7	Var 8	Var 9	Var 10	Var 11	Var 12	Var 13	Var 14
1	0													
2	8	0												
3	7	2	0											
4	5	4	5	0										
5	8	5	4	6	0									
6	7	5	6	6	8	0								
7	4	5	6	3	7	4	0							
8	8	5	4	6	3	8	7	0						
9	3	7	9	4	8	7	5	8	0					
10	5	6	7	6	9	4	4	9	6	0				
11	9	5	4	6	3	8	7	3	8	9	0			
12	9	4	3	7	5	7	7	5	8	9	5	0		
13	4	6	6	3	7	5	4	8	4	5	7	7	0	
14	6	6	7	6	8	2	4	9	7	3	9	7	5	0

The matrix with mean scores can be considered as one by one distances between all of the medicines connected with one another by straight lines in 14 different ways. Already more and less similar drugs can directly be read from the matrix. But more precision is desired. Along an x- and y-axis they are subsequently modeled using the equation: the distance between drug i and drug j = $\sqrt{[(x_i - x_j)^2 + (y_i - y_j)^2]}$. SPSS statistical software will be used for analysis. Start by opening the data file in your SPSS mounted computer.

Command

Analyze….Scale….Multidimensional scaling (PROXSCAL)….Data Format: click The data are proximities….Number of Sources: click One matrix source…. One Source: click The proximities are in a matrix across columns….click Define…. enter all variables (medicines) into "Proximities"….Model: Shape: click Lower-triangular matrix….Proximity Transformation: click Interval…. Dimensions: Minimum: enter 2….Maximum: enter 2….click Continue….click Plots….mark Common space….mark Transformed proximities versus distances….click Continue ….click: Output….mark Common space coordinates….mark Multiple stress measures….click Continue….click OK.

The underneath table are in the output.

Stress and Fit Measures

Normalized Raw Stress	,00819
Stress-I	,09051[a]
Stress-II	,21640[a]
S-Stress	,02301[b]
Dispersion Accounted For (D.A.F.)	,99181
Tucker's Coefficient of Congruence	,99590

PROXSCAL minimizes Normalized Raw Stress.

a. Optimal scaling factor = 1,008.

b. Optimal scaling factor = ,995.

The output sheet also gives the uncertainty of the model (stress = standard error) and dispersion values. The model is assumed to appropriately describe the data if they are respectively < 0.20 and approximately 1.0.

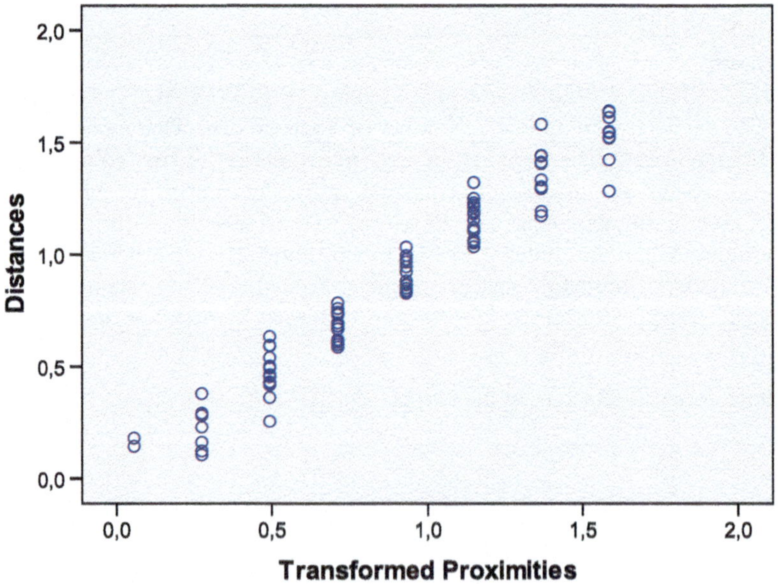

The above graph of the actual distances as observed versus the distances fitted by the statistical program is given. The actual proximities plotted ordinally are plotted against the best fit linear transformation computed by the statistical program. A perfect fit should produce a straight line, a poor fit produces a lot of spread around a line or even no line at all. The figure is not perfect, but it shows a very good fit as expected from the stress and fit measures.

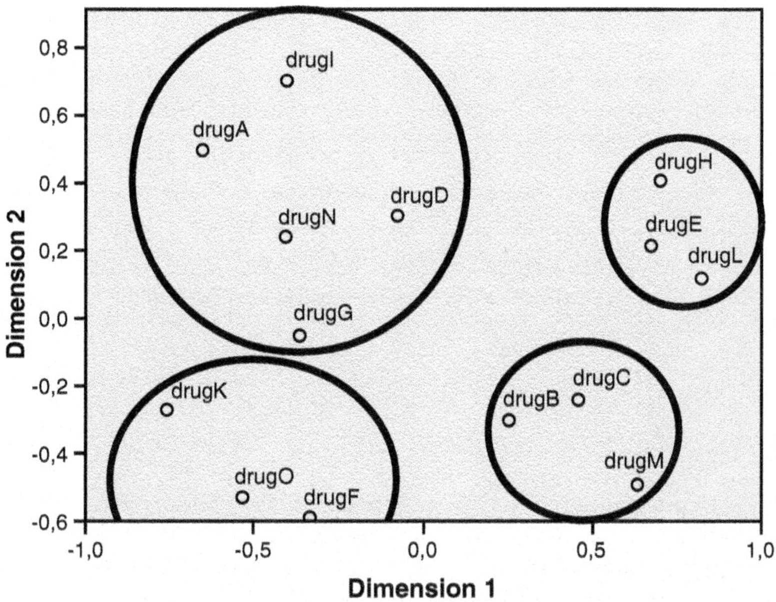

Finally, the above figure is given, and shows the most important part of the outcome. The standardized x- and y-axes values give some insight in the relative position of the medicines according to perception of our study population. Four clusters are identified. Using Microsoft's drawing commands we can encircle the clusters as identified. The cluster at the upper right quadrant comprises high priorities of the patients along both the x- an the y-axis. The cluster at the lower left quadrant comprises low priorities of the patients along both axes. If, pharmacologically, the drugs in the right upper quadrant were highly potent with little side effects, then the patients' priorities would fairly match the pharmacological properties of the medicines.

11.3.2 Preference Scaling

The example from the above traditional efficacy analysis section will be used once more. In a prospective study of preference ranking of the 15 pain killers, 42 patients were tested 15 times in a randomized crossover setting. Part of the data file is underneath Var = variable).

Var 1	2	3	4	5	6	7	8	9	10	11	12	13	14	15
12	13	7	4	5	2	8	10	11	14	3	1	6	9	15
14	11	6	3	10	4	15	8	9	12	7	1	5	2	13
13	10	12	14	3	2	9	8	7	11	1	6	4	5	15
7	14	11	3	6	8	12	10	9	15	4	1	2	5	13
14	9	6	15	13	2	11	8	7	10	12	1	3	4	5
9	11	15	4	7	6	14	10	8	12	5	2	3	1	13
9	14	5	6	8	4	13	11	12	15	7	2	1	3	10
15	10	12	6	8	2	13	9	7	11	3	1	5	4	14
13	12	2	4	5	8	10	11	3	15	7	9	6	1	14
15	13	10	7	6	4	9	11	12	14	5	2	8	1	3
9	2	4	13	8	5	1	10	6	7	11	15	14	12	3

Var 1–15 preference scores (1 = most prefered, 15 = least prefered)

Only the first 11 patients are given. The entire data file is entitled "prefscal" and is in extras.springer.com.

To 42 patients 15 different pain-killers are administered, and the patients are requested to rank them in order of preference from 1 "most prefered" to 15 "least prefered".

We will try and draw a three dimensional view of the individually assigned preferences. We will use SPSS 19.0. Start by opening the data file.

Command

Graphs....Legacy Dialogs....3-D Bar....X-axis represents: click Separate variables....Z-axis represents: click Individual cases....Define....Bars Represent: enter pain-killers 1-15....Show Cases on: click Y-axis....Show Cases with: click Case number....click OK.

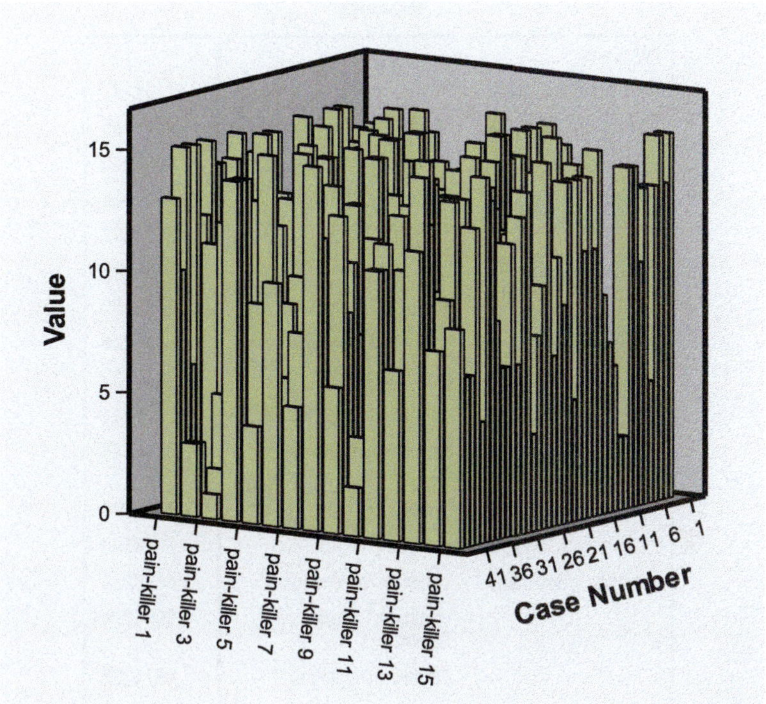

The above figure shows the result: a very irregular pattern consisting of multiple areas with either high or low preference is observed. We will now perform a preference scaling analysis. Like with proximity scaling, preference assessments is mapped in a 2 dimensional plane with the rank orders of the medicines as measures of distance between the medicines. Two types of maps are constructed: an aggregate map giving average distances of the entire population or individual maps of single patients, and an ideal point map where ideal points have to be interpreted as a map with ideal medicines, one for each patient. SPSS 19.0 is used once more.

Command

Analyze....Scale....Multidimensional Unfolding (PREFSCAL)....enter all variables (medicines) into "Proximities"....click Model....click Dissimilarities.... Dimensions: Minimum enter 2 ....Maximum enter 2....Proximity Transformations: click Ordinal ....click Within each row separately....click Continue.... click Options: imputation by: enter Spearman....click Continue....click Plots: mark Final common space....click Continue....click Output: mark Fit measures ....mark Final common space....click Continue....click OK.

Measures

Iterations		115
Final Function Value		,7104127
Function Value Parts	Stress Part	,2563298
	Penalty Part	1,9688939
Badness of Fit	Normalized Stress	,0651568
	Kruskal's Stress-I	,2552582
	Kruskal's Stress-II	,6430926
	Young's S-Stress-I	,3653360
	Young's S-Stress-II	,5405226
Goodness of Fit	Dispersion Accounted For	,9348432
	Variance Accounted For	,7375011
	Recovered Preference Orders	,7804989
	Spearman's Rho	,8109694
	Kendall's Tau-b	,6816390
Variation Coefficients	Variation Proximities	,5690984
	Variation Transformed Proximities	,5995274
	Variation Distances	,4674236
Degeneracy Indices	Sum-of-Squares of DeSarbo's Intermixedness Indices	,2677061
	Shepard's Rough Nondegeneracy Index	,7859410

The above table gives the stress (standard error) and fit measures. The best fit distances as estimated by the model are adequate: measures of stress including normalized stress and Kruskal's stress-I are close to 0.20 or less, the value of dispersion measures (Dispersion Accounted For) is close to 1.0. The table also shows whether there is a risk of a *degenerate* solution, otherwise called loss function. The individual proximities have a tendency to form circles, and when averaged for obtaining average proximities, there is a tendency for the average treatment places to center in the middle of the map. The solution is a penalty term, but in our example we need not worry. The DeSarbo's and Shepard criteria are close to respectively 0 and 80%, and no penalty adjustment is required.

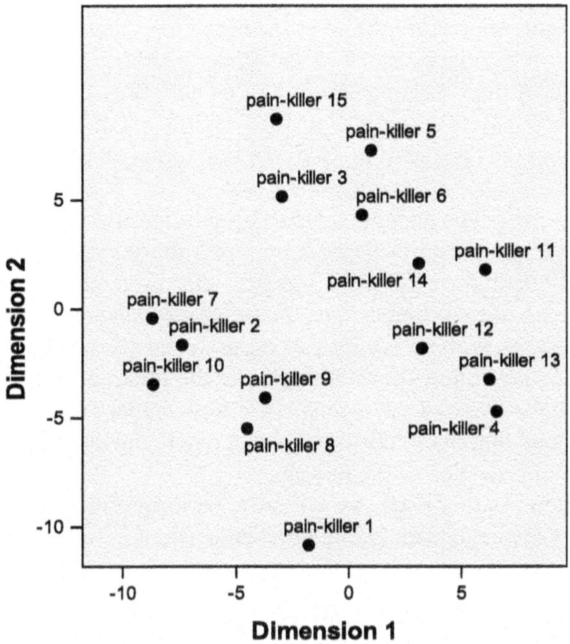
pain-killer 15
pain-killer 5
pain-killer 3
pain-killer 6
pain-killer 11
pain-killer 14
pain-killer 7
pain-killer 2
pain-killer 12
pain-killer 10
pain-killer 13
pain-killer 9
pain-killer 4
pain-killer 8
pain-killer 1
Dimension 2
5
0
-5
-10
-10
-5
0
5
Dimension 1

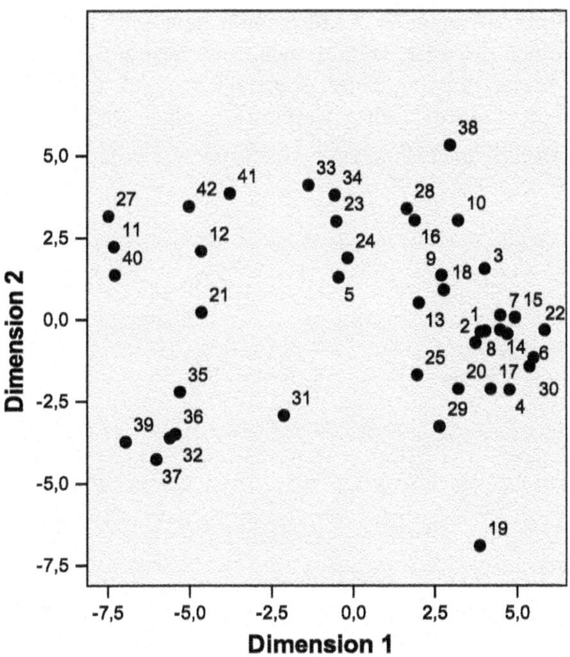
38
33 34
41
42
28
27
23
10
11
12
24
16
40
9
3
18
21
5
7 15
22
13
1
2
8 14
6
25
35
20 17
30
31
4
29
39
36
32
37
19
Dimension 2
5,0
2,5
0,0
-2,5
-5,0
-7,5
-7,5
-5,0
-2,5
0,0
2,5
5,0
Dimension 1

The above figure (upper graph) gives the most important part of the output. The standardized x- and y-axes values of the upper graph give some insight in the relative position of the medicines according to our study population. The results can be understood as the relative position of the medicines according to the perception of our study population. Both the horizontal and the vertical dimension appears to discriminate between different preferences. The lower graph gives the patients' *ideal points*. The patients seem to be split into two clusters with different preferences, although with much variation along the y-axis. The dense cluster in the right lower quadrant represented patients with preferences both along the x- and y-axis. Instead of two-dimensions, multidimensional scaling enables to assess multiple dimensions each of which can be assigned to one particular cause for proximity. This may sound speculative, but if the pharmacological properties of the drugs match the place of the medicines in a particular dimension, then we will be more convinced that the multi-dimensional display gives, indeed, an important insight in the real priorities of the patients.

In order to address this issue, we will now perform a multidimensional scaling procedure of the above data including three dimensions.

Command

Analyze….Scale….Multidimensional Unfolding (PREFSCAL)….enter all variables (medicines) into "Proximities"….click Model….click Dissimilarities…. Dimensions: Minimum enter 3 ….Maximum enter 3….Proximity Transformations: click Ordinal ….click Within each row separately….click Continue…. click Options: imputation by: enter Spearman….click Continue….click Plots: mark Final common space….click Continue….click Output: mark Fit measures ….mark Final common space….click Continue….click OK.

Final Column Coordinates

Painkiller no.	Dimension 1	2	3
1	-2.49	-9.08	-4.55
2	-7.08	-1.81	1.43
3	-3.46	3.46	-2.81
4	5.41	-4.24	1.67
5	-.36	6.21	5.25
6	.17	1.88	-3.27
7	-7.80	-2.07	-1.59
8	-5.17	-4.18	2.91
9	4.75	-.59	4.33
10	-6.80	-4.83	.27
11	6.22	2.50	.88
12	3.71	-1.27	-.49
13	5.30	-2.95	1.51
14	2.82	1.66	-2.09
15	-4.35	2.76	-6.72

The output sheets shows the standardized mean preference values of the different pain-killers as x- y-, and z-axis coordinates. The best fit outcome of the three-dimensional (3-D) model can be visualized in a 3-D figure. SPSS 19.0 is used. First cut and paste the data from the above table to the preference scaling file or another file. Then proceed.

Command

Graphs. . . .Legacy Dialogs. . . .Scatter/Dot. . . .click 3-D Scatter. . . .click Define. . . . Y-Axis: enter dimension 1. . . .X-Axis: enter dimension 2. . . .Z-Axis: enter dimension 3. . . .click OK.

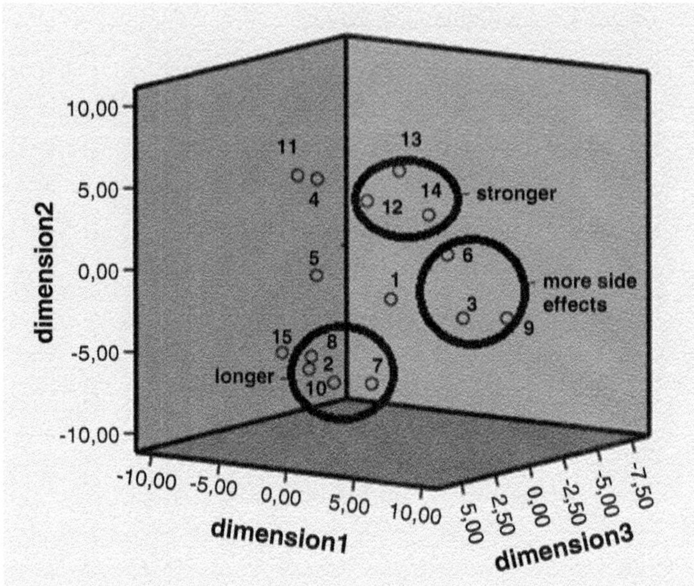

The above figure gives the best fit outcome of a 3-dimensional scaling model. Three clusters were identified, consistent with patients' preferences along an x-, y-, and z-axis. Using Microsoft's drawing commands we can encircle the clusters as identified. In the figure an example is given of how pharmacological properties could be used to explain the cluster pattern.

11.4 Discussion

Multidimensional scaling is helpful and better sensitive than traditional t-tests, both to underscore the pharmacological properties of the medicines under studies, and to identify, what effects are really important to patients, and uses for these purposes estimated proximities as surrogates for counted estimates of patients' opinions.

Multidimensional scaling can, like regression analysis, be used two ways, (1) for estimating preferences of treatment modalities in a population, (2) for assessing the preferred treatment modalities in individual patients.

In this chapter the traditional efficacy analysis consisted of confidence intervals, paired t-tests, equivalence testing, and the machine learning analyses included multidimensional scaling. The machine learning analyses provided better sensitivity of testing, and were more informative.

11.5 References

To readers requesting more background, theoretical and mathematical information of computations given, several textbooks complementary to the current production and written by the same authors are available:

Statistics applied to clinical studies 5th edition, 2012,
Machine learning in medicine a complete overview, 2015,
SPSS for starters and 2nd levelers 2nd edition, 2015,
Clinical data analysis on a pocket calculator 2nd edition, 2016,
Understanding clinical data analysis from published research, 2016,
Modern meta-analysis, 2017,
Regression analysis in clinical research, 2018,
Modern Bayesian statistics in clinical research, 2018.
The Analysis of Safety Data of Drug Trials, an Update, 2019.

All of them have been edited by Springer Heidelberg Germany.

Chapter 12
Binary Decision-Trees for Efficacy Analysis

Contents

Abstract In a 1004 patient random sample, the effects of age, cholesterol levels, smoking levels, education levels, and weight levels on infarct rating was tested, both traditionally, and with the help of machine learning.

Traditional efficacy analysis consisted of
discretization of continuous predictors,
crosstabs with chi-square statistics.

Machine learning efficacy analysis consisted of binary decision-tree methods.

The machine learning methods provided better sensitivity of testing, and were more informative.

Keywords Clinical trials · Traditional efficacy analysis · Machine learning efficacy analysis · Binary decision-tree methods

12.1 Introduction

The effects of risk factors on health risks can be analyzed with chi-squares, if the outcome is binary or with T-tests and analyses of variance, if continuous. However, in order to obtain a more precise information of the magnitude of the effects of various predictors in various subclasses decision trees is a relevant method. Also extended mark-up language files can be constructed for predicting probabilities of a data outcome through regression trees with the help of so-called exhaustive search.

T. J. Cleophas, A. H. Zwinderman, *Efficacy Analysis in Clinical Trials an Update*,
https://doi.org/10.1007/978-3-030-19918-0_12

In Sect. 1.12, Chap. 1, the use of regression analyses for efficacy analyses is discussed, and in Sect. 1.13 the use of clinical trials for the assessment of causal health effects of factors other than medicines is discussed. For example, effects of interventions like angioplasties, surgeries, renal transplants etc. Many more factors can be tested in clinical trials, for example,

age factors
psychological factors
social factors
physical factors
economical factors,
and, any factor with a supposedly causal effect on health or sickness.

In this chapter traditional efficacy analysis will be tested against a machine learning methodology entitled binary decision trees. The traditional efficacy analysis will consist of discretized continuous predictors, and crosstabs with chi-square statistics.

12.2 Data Example with Binary Outcome

In 1004 patients the effect of age, cholesterol level, smoking, education, and body weight level, on the risk of infarction was studied (Var = variable).

Var 1	Var 2	Var 3	Var 4	Var 5	Var 6
,00	44,86	1,00	,00	1,00	2,00
,00	42,71	2,00	,00	1,00	2,00
,00	43,34	3,00	,00	2,00	2,00
,00	44,02	3,00	,00	1,00	2,00
,00	67,97	1,00	,00	2,00	2,00
,00	40,31	2,00	,00	2,00	2,00
,00	66,56	1,00	,00	2,00	2,00
,00	45,95	1,00	,00	2,00	2,00
,00	52,27	1,00	,00	1,00	2,00
,00	43,86	1,00	,00	1,00	2,00
,00	46,58	3,00	,00	2,00	1,00
,00	53,83	2,00	,00	2,00	2,00
,00	49,48	1,00	,00	2,00	1,00

Var 1 infarct_rating (,00 no, 1,00 yes)
Var 2 age (years)
Var 3 cholesterol_level (1,00–3,00)
Var 4 smoking (,00 no, 1,00 yes)
Var 5 education (levels 1,00 and 2,00)
Var 6 weight_level (levels 1,00 and 2,00)

The data from the first 13 patients are shown only. See extras.springer.com for the entire data file entitled "decisiontreebinary".

Except for the variable age, all variables were discrete. For traditional efficacy analysis this variable will first be transformed into a discrete one. Start by opening the data file in the SPSS statistical software program of your computer. Command.

Command
Analyze. . . .Descriptives. . . .Var(s): enter age. . . .click OK.

Descriptive Statistics

	N	Minimum	Maximum	Mean	Std. Deviation
Age	1004	40,02	82,45	55,0430	8,60676
Valid N (listwise)	1004				

The above output shows that 55 years is mean age, and we will take 55 as cut-off for a novel variable entitled age level.

Command
Transform. . . .Compute Variable. . . .Target Variable: type agelevel. . . .Numeric Expression: enter age. . . .enter from the blue square of the screen ">". . . .then enter "55". . . .click OK.

In the data screen now a novel variable has been added entitled agelevel.

12.3 Traditional Efficacy Analysis

Next, the effect of all of the predictors of the health risk was assessed with Pearson chi-square tests. Command.

Command
Analyze. . . .Descriptive Statistics. . . .Crosstabs. . . .Row(s): cholesterol level. . . . Column(s): infarct rating. . . .Statistics. . . .mark Chi-square. . . .click Continue. . . . click OK.

The first two tables underneath are in the output sheets.

cholesterol level * infarct rating Crosstabulation

Count

		infarct rating		Total
		no	yes	
cholesterol level	Low	89	49	138
	Medium	86	365	451
	High	32	383	415
Total		207	797	1004

Chi-Square Tests

	Value	df	Asymp. Sig. (2-sided)
Pearson Chi-Square	205,214[a]	2	,000
Likelihood Ratio	177,274	2	,000
Linear-by-Linear Association	166,773	1	,000
N of Valid Cases	1004		

a. 0 cells (,0%) have expected count less than 5. The minimum expected count is 28,45.

The above tables show, that cholesterol level is a very significant predictor of infatc rating. The same procedure is performed with all of the other predictor variables.

smoking * infarct rating Crosstabulation

Count

		infarct rating		Total
		no	yes	
smoking	no	189	417	606
	yes	18	378	396
	2,00	0	2	2
Total		207	797	1004

Chi-Square Tests

	Value	df	Asymp. Sig. (2-sided)
Pearson Chi-Square	104,391[a]	2	,000
Likelihood Ratio	123,150	2	,000
Linear-by-Linear Association	103,705	1	,000
N of Valid Cases	1004		

a. 2 cells (33,3%) have expected count less than 5. The minimum expected count is ,41.

education * infarct rating Crosstabulation

Count

		infarct rating		Total
		no	yes	
education	High school	100	392	492
	College	107	405	512
Total		207	797	1004

Chi-Square Tests

	Value	df	Asymp. Sig. (2-sided)	Exact Sig. (2-sided)	Exact Sig. (1-sided)
Pearson Chi-Square	,050[a]	1	,822		
Continuity Correction[b]	,021	1	,884		
Likelihood Ratio	,050	1	,822		
Fisher's Exact Test				,876	,442
Linear-by-Linear Association	,050	1	,823		
N of Valid Cases	1004				

a. 0 cells (,0%) have expected count less than 5. The minimum expected count is 101,44.
b. Computed only for a 2x2 table

weight level * infarct rating Crosstabulation

Count

		infarct rating		Total
		no	yes	
weight level	normal	30	394	424
	high	177	403	580
Total		207	797	1004

Chi-Square Tests

	Value	df	Asymp. Sig. (2-sided)	Exact Sig. (2-sided)	Exact Sig. (1-sided)
Pearson Chi-Square	82,239[a]	1	,000		
Continuity Correction[b]	80,813	1	,000		
Likelihood Ratio	91,410	1	,000		
Fisher's Exact Test				,000	,000
Linear-by-Linear Association	82,157	1	,000		
N of Valid Cases	1004				

a. 0 cells (,0%) have expected count less than 5. The minimum expected count is 87,42.
b. Computed only for a 2x2 table

agelevel * infarct rating Crosstabulation

Count

		infarct rating		Total
		no	yes	
agelevel	,00	174	422	596
	1,00	33	375	408
Total		207	797	1004

Chi-Square Tests

	Value	df	Asymp. Sig. (2-sided)	Exact Sig. (2-sided)	Exact Sig. (1-sided)
Pearson Chi-Square	65,923[a]	1	,000		
Continuity Correction[b]	64,640	1	,000		
Likelihood Ratio	72,699	1	,000		
Fisher's Exact Test				,000	,000
Linear-by-Linear Association	65,858	1	,000		
N of Valid Cases	1004				

a. 0 cells (,0%) have expected count less than 5. The minimum expected count is 84,12.
b. Computed only for a 2x2 table

Except for the predictor education level, all of the above chi-square tests of predictors on infarct risks were very significant,. However, the univariate tests did not account possible confoundings and interactions. A multiple logistic regression was performed. Command.

Command
Analyze. . . .Regression. . . .Binary logistic. . . .Dependent: infarct rating. . . . Covariates: cholesterol level, smoking, education, weight level, agelevel. . . . click OK.

A multiple binary logistic regression including all of the predictors simultaneously showed, that all of the predictors, except again education level were independent determinants of the risk of infarction, and so, cholesterol levels remained statistically significant even adjusted for the effects of agelevel and weight level (type I error 0.10).

Variables in the Equation

		B	S.E.	Wald	df	Sig.	Exp(B)
Step 1[a]	cholesterol_level	1,591	,151	110,426	1	,000	4,911
	smoking	1,958	,357	30,029	1	,000	7,086
	education	-,066	,194	,117	1	,732	,936
	weight_level	-,538	,312	2,977	1	,084	,584
	agelevel	1,579	,232	46,383	1	,000	4,852
	Constant	-1,909	,736	6,725	1	,010	,148

a. Variable(s) entered on step 1: cholesterol_level, smoking, education, weight_level, agelevel.

According to the above table the patients with high cholesterol levels will have approximately 5 times higher risk of infarction, than those with low cholesterol. Those with smoking 7 times higher, and those with high age 4.8 times higher. If you have at the same time (1) a high cholesterol, have been (1) a smoker, and have (3) a high age, then your risk of infarction will be about $5 \times 7 \times 4.8 \approx 168$ times higher than the risk you would have had without all of these risk factors. This is of course a pretty crude approach, and somewhat unrealistic result. Cholesterol abusers may have a higher risk of abusing other risk factors like smoking, and, so, many interactions may not have been covered in the above analysis. In order to obtain a more precise information about the magnitude of the effects of the various predictors in various subclasses of the data decision tree analysis may be a relevant method. If you additionally make use of a training sample, you may obtain even better precision.

12.4 Decision-Trees for Efficacy Analysis

Decision trees are, so-called, non-metric or non-algorithmic methods adequate for fitting nominal and interval data (the latter either categorical or continuous). Better accuracy from decision trees is sometimes obtained by the use of a training sample. This chapter is to assess, whether decision trees can be appropriately applied to predict health risks. Also will be assessed whether decision trees can be trained to predict in individual future patients risk of infarction, and ldl (low density lipoprotein) cholesterol decrease. The above data file will be used once again.

In the 1004 patient data file of risk factors for myocardial infarct a so-called chi-squared automatic interaction (CHAID) model is used for analysis. Also an XML (eXtended Markup Language) will be exported for the analysis of future data. Start by opening the data file in your computer mounted with SPSS.

Command

Click Transform....click Random Number Generators....click Set Starting Point.... click Fixed Value (2000000)....click OK....click Classify....Tree.... Dependent Variable: enter infarct rating....Independent Variables: enter age, cholesterol level, smoking, education, weight level....Growing Method: select CHAID....click Categories: Target mark yes....Continue....click Output: mark Tree in table format....Criteria: Parent Node type 200, Child Node type 100.... click Continue.... click Save: mark Terminal node number, Predicted probabilities.... in Export Tree Model as XML mark Training sample....click Browse........in File name enter "exportdecisiontreebinary" ....in Look in: enter the appropriate map in your computer for storage....click Save....click OK.

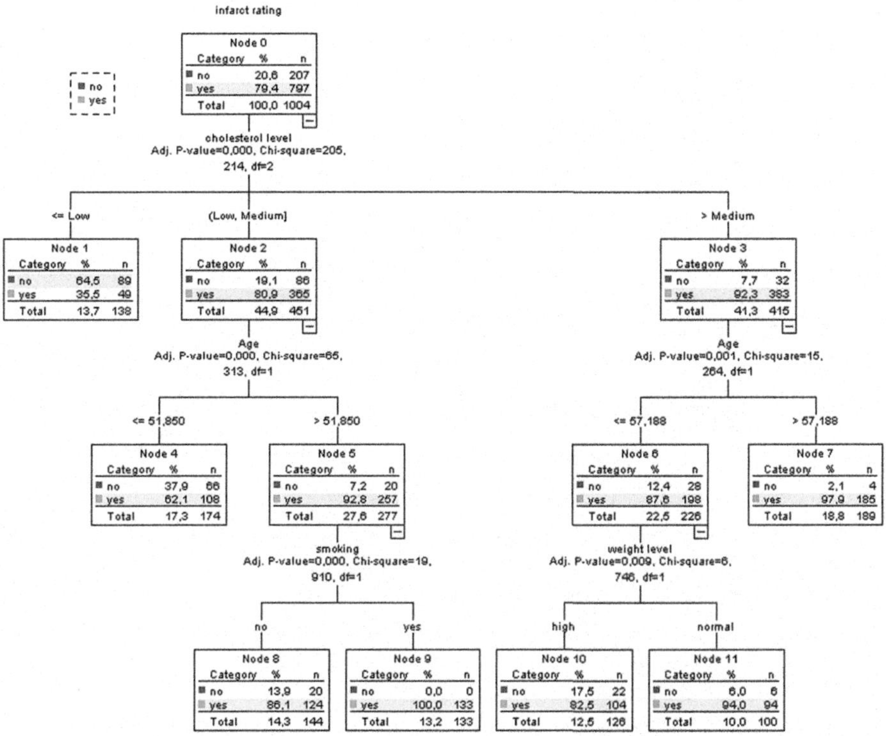

The output sheets show the decision tree and various tables. The Cholesterol level is the best predictor of the infarct rating. For low cholesterol the cholesterol level is the only significant predictor of infarction: only 35.5 % will have an infarction. In the medium and high cholesterol groups age is the next best predictor. In the elderly with medium cholesterol smoking contributes considerably to the risk of infarction. In contrast, in the younger with high cholesterol those with normal weight are slightly more at risk of infarction than those with high weights. For each node (subgroup) the number of cases, the chi-square value, and level of significance is given. A p-value < 0.05 indicates that the difference between the 2 × 2 or 3 × 2 tables of the paired nodes are significantly different from one another. All of the p-values were very significant.

The risk and classification tables indicate, that the category infarction predicted by the model is wrong in 0.166 = 16.6% of the cases (underneath table). A correct prediction of 83.4 % is fine. However, in those without an infarction no infarction is predicted in only 43.0% of the cases (underneath table).

Risk

Estimate	Std. Error
,166	,012

Growing Method: CHAID
Dependent Variable: infarct rating

Classification

Observed	Predicted		
	no	yes	Percent Correct
no	89	118	43,0%
yes	49	748	93,9%
Overall Percentage	13,7%	86,3%	83,4%

Growing Method: CHAID
Dependent Variable: infarct rating

When returning to the original data file we will observe 3 new variables, (1) the terminal node number, (2) the predicted probabilities of no infarction for each case, (3) the predicted probabilities of yes infarction for each case. In a binary logistic regression it can be tested, that the latter variables are much better predictors of the probability of infarction than each of the original variables are. The saved XML file will now be used to compute the predicted PAF rate in 6 novel patients with the following characteristics. For convenience the XML file is given in extras.springer.com.

Var 2	Var 3	Var 4	Var 5	Var 6
59,16	2,00	,00	1,00	2,00
53,42	1,00	,00	2,00	2,00
43,02	2,00	,00	2,00	2,00
76,91	3,00	1,00	1,00	1,00
70,53	2,00	,00	1,00	2,00
47,02	3,00	1,00	1,00	1,00

Var 2 age (years)
Var 3 cholesterol_level (1,00–3,00)
Var 4 smoking (,00 no, 1,00 yes)
Var 5 education (level 1,00 and 2,00)
Var 6 weight_level (1,00 and 2,00)

Enter the above data in a new SPSS data file.

Command

Utilities....click Scoring Wizard....click Browse....click Select....Folder: enter the exportdecisiontreebinary.xml file....click Select....in Scoring Wizard click Next....mark Node Number....mark Probability of Predicted Category....click Next....click Finish.

The above data file now gives the individual predicted nodes numbers and probabilities of infarct for the six novel patients as computed by the linear model with the help of the XML file. Enter the above data in a new SPSS data file.

Var 2	Var 3	Var 4	Var 5	Var 6	Var 7	Var 8
59,16	2,00	,00	1,00	2,00	8,00	,86
53,42	1,00	,00	2,00	2,00	1,00	,64
43,02	2,00	,00	2,00	2,00	4,00	,62
76,91	3,00	1,00	1,00	1,00	7,00	,98
70,53	2,00	,00	1,00	2,00	8,00	,86
47,02	3,00	1,00	1,00	1,00	11,00	,94

Var 2 age
Var 3 cholesterol_level
Var 4 smoking
Var 5 education
Var 6 weight_level
Var 7 predicted node number
Var 8 predicted probability of infarct

The Decision-Tree procedure provided valuable information additional to the traditional efficacy analysis, and predicting probabilities of the outcome of future patients from an XML (Extended Markup Language) file of the old data is another possibility not available with traditional methods.

12.5 Discussion

The effects of risk factors on health risks can be analyzed with chi-squares if the outcome is binary or with T-tests and analyses of variance if continuous. However, in order to obtain a more precise information of the magnitude of the effects of various predictors in various subclasses decision trees is a relevant method. Also extended mark-up language files can be constructed for predicting probabilities of a data outcome through regression trees with the help of so-called exhaustive search.

In the current chapter decision trees with binary outcomes are tested against traditional efficacy analyses with chi-square tests. The binary decision tree models provided better sensitivity of testing with multiple risk and classification tables all of whom have been statistically tested. In addition, a trained XML file was produced, enabling to make predictions of future patients.

In this chapter the traditional efficacy analysis consisted of discretized continuous predictors, and crosstabs with chi-square statistics, and the machine learning analyses included binary decision tree methodologies. The machine learning analyses provided better sensitivity of testing, and were more informative.

12.6 References

To readers requesting more background, theoretical and mathematical information of computations given, several textbooks complementary to the current production and written by the same authors are available:

Statistics applied to clinical studies 5th edition, 2012,
Machine learning in medicine a complete overview, 2015,
SPSS for starters and 2nd levelers 2nd edition, 2015,
Clinical data analysis on a pocket calculator 2nd edition, 2016,
Understanding clinical data analysis from published research, 2016,
Modern meta-analysis, 2017,
Regression analysis in clinical research, 2018,
Modern Bayesian statistics in clinical research, 2018.
The Analysis of Safety Data of Drug Trials, an Update, 2019.

All of them have been edited by Springer Heidelberg Germany.

Chapter 13
Continuous Decision-Trees for Efficacy Analysis

Contents

Abstract In a 953 patient random sample the effect of weight reduction, gender, sport, medical treatments, and diet on ldl cholesterol reduction was tested, both traditionally, and with the help of machine learning.

Traditional efficacy analysis was composed of

one-way analyses of variance (anova),

multiple linear regressions.

Machine learning efficacy analysis was composed of continuous decision-tree methods.

The machine learning methods provided better sensitivity of testing, and were more informative.

Keywords Clinical trials · Traditional efficacy analysis · Machine learning efficacy analysis · Continuous decision-tree methods

13.1 Introduction

The effects of risk factors on health risks can be analyzed with chi-squares, if the outcome is binary or with T-tests and analyses of variance, if continuous. However, in order to obtain a more precise information of the magnitude of the effects of various predictors in various subclasses decision trees is a relevant method. Also extended mark-up language files can be constructed for predicting probabilities of a data outcome through regression trees with the help of so-called exhaustive search.

T. J. Cleophas, A. H. Zwinderman, *Efficacy Analysis in Clinical Trials an Update*,
https://doi.org/10.1007/978-3-030-19918-0_13

In Sect. 1.12, Chap. 1, the use of regression analyses for efficacy analyses is discussed, and in Sect. 1.13 the use of clinical trials for the assessment of causal health effects of factors other than medicines is discussed. For example, effects of interventions like angioplasties, surgeries, renal transplants etc. Many more factors can be tested in clinical trials, for example,

age factors
psychological factors
social factors
physical factors
economical factors,
and, any factor with a supposedly causal effect on health or sickness.

In this chapter traditional efficacy analysis will be tested against a machine learning methodology entitled continuous decision trees. The traditional efficacy analysis will consist of one-way analyses of variance, and multiple linear regressions.

13.2 Data Example with Continuous Outcome (Var = Variable)

Var 1	Var 2	Var 3	Var 4	Var 5	Var 6
3,41	0	1	3,00	3	0
1,86	−1	1	2,00	3	1
,85	−2	1	1,00	4	1
1,63	−1	1	2,00	3	1
6,84	4	0	4,00	2	0
1,00	−2	0	1,00	3	0
1,14	−2	1	1,00	3	1
2,97	0	1	3,00	4	0
1,05	−2	1	1,00	4	1
,63	−2	0	1,00	3	0
1,18	−2	0	1,00	2	0
,96	−2	1	1,00	2	0
8,28	5	0	4,00	2	1

Var 1 ldl_reduction (outcome)
Var 2 weight_redcution
Var 3 gender
Var 4 sport
Var 5 treatment_level
Var 6 diet

For the decision tree with continuous outcome the classification and regression tree (CRT) model can be applied, but first a traditional efficacy analysis will be performed. A 953 patient data file is used of various predictors of ldl (low-density-lipoprotein)-cholesterol reduction including weight reduction, gender, sport, treatment level, diet. The data file is in extras.springer.com, and is entitled "decisiontreecontinuous".

13.3 Traditional Efficacy Analysis

For traditional efficacy analysis one way analyses of variance were performed with various predictors and the ldl cholesterol reduction as outcome. Start by opening the data file in your computer loaded with SPSS statistical software. Command.

Command
Analyze....Compare Means....One Way ANOVA....Dependent List: ldl reduction.... Factor: weight reduction....click OK.

The underneath table is in the output. It shows, that weight reduction is a very significant predictor of ldl (low density lipoprotein cholesterol) reduction.

ANOVA

ldl reduction

	Sum of Squares	df	Mean Square	F	Sig.
Between Groups	4438,460	463	9,586	361,083	,000
Within Groups	12,982	489	,027		
Total	4451,443	952			

Similarly, more one by one one-way anovas were performed, and results are given below.

ANOVA

ldl reduction

	Sum of Squares	df	Mean Square	F	Sig.
Between Groups	6,246	1	6,246	1,336	,248
Within Groups	4445,197	951	4,674		
Total	4451,443	952			

by genders

ANOVA

ldl reduction

	Sum of Squares	df	Mean Square	F	Sig.
Between Groups	3718,038	3	1239,346	1603,670	,000
Within Groups	733,405	949	,773		
Total	4451,443	952			

by sports

ANOVA

ldl reduction

	Sum of Squares	df	Mean Square	F	Sig.
Between Groups	92,488	4	23,122	5,029	,001
Within Groups	4358,955	948	4,598		
Total	4451,443	952			

by treatments

ANOVA

ldl reduction

	Sum of Squares	df	Mean Square	F	Sig.
Between Groups	3,638	1	3,638	,778	,378
Within Groups	4447,805	951	4,677		
Total	4451,443	952			

by diet

With ldl cholesterol reduction as outcome variable and weight, reduction, gender, sport, treatment, and diet as determinants, the univariate analyses produced several very significant effects. Particularly, weight reductions, sports, treatments were very significant independent determinants of ldl cholesterol reductions. However, interactions and confounders were not accounted.

Instead of one way anova (analysis of variance), a multiple linear regression with ldl cholesterol reduction as outcome and all of the above determinants as predictors is possible.

Command

Analyze. . . .Regression. . . .Linear. . . .Dependent: enter ldl reduction. . . .Independent(s): enter weight reduction, gender, sport, treatment level. . . .diet. . . .click OK.

Model Summary

Model	R	R Square	Adjusted R Square	Std. Error of the Estimate
1	,986[a]	,972	,972	,36045

a. Predictors: (Constant), diet, treatment level, gender, weight reduction, sport

ANOVA[b]

Model		Sum of Squares	df	Mean Square	F	Sig.
1	Regression	4328,402	5	865,680	6662,847	,000[a]
	Residual	123,040	947	,130		
	Total	4451,443	952			

a. Predictors: (Constant), diet, treatment level, gender, weight reduction, sport
b. Dependent Variable: ldl reduction

Coefficients[a]

Model		Unstandardized Coefficients		Standardized Coefficients	t	Sig.
		B	Std. Error	Beta		
1	(Constant)	2,786	,065		43,088	,000
	weight reduction	,985	,012	,944	81,937	,000
	gender	-,015	,023	-,003	-,633	,527
	sport	,095	,023	,047	4,060	,000
	treatment level	,009	,010	,005	,954	,340
	diet	-,017	,023	-,004	-,716	,474

a. Dependent Variable: ldl reduction

The multiple linear regression showed, that weight reduction and sport were very significant independent determinants of the outcome ldl cholesterol reduction. However, the other three predictors (including treatments) were now insignificant. In order to obtain a more precise information about the magnitude of the effects of the various predictors in various subclasses of the data, decision tree analysis may be a relevant method. If you, additionally, make use of a training sample, you may obtain even better precision.

13.4 Decision-Tree for Efficacy Analysis

For the decision tree with continuous outcome the classification and regression tree (CRT) model can be applied. The above 953 patient data file of various predictors of ldl (low-density-lipoprotein)-cholesterol reduction including weight reduction, gender, sport, treatment level, diet is used once more. The data file is in extras.springer.com, and is entitled "decisiontreecontinuous". The data file is opened in your computer.

Command

Click Transform….click Random Number Generators….click Set Starting Point…. click Fixed Value (2000000)….click OK….click Analyze…. Classify…Tree…. Dependent Variable: enter ldl_reduction…. Independent Variables: enter weight reduction, gender, sport, treatment level, diet….Growing Methods: select CRT ….click Criteria: enter Parent Node 300, Child Node 100….click Output: Tree mark Tree in table format….click Continue….click Save….mark Terminal node number….mark Predicted value….in Export Tree Model as XML mark Training sample….click Browse……..in File name enter "exportdecisiontreecontinuous" ….in Look in: enter the appropriate map in your computer for storage….click Save….click OK.

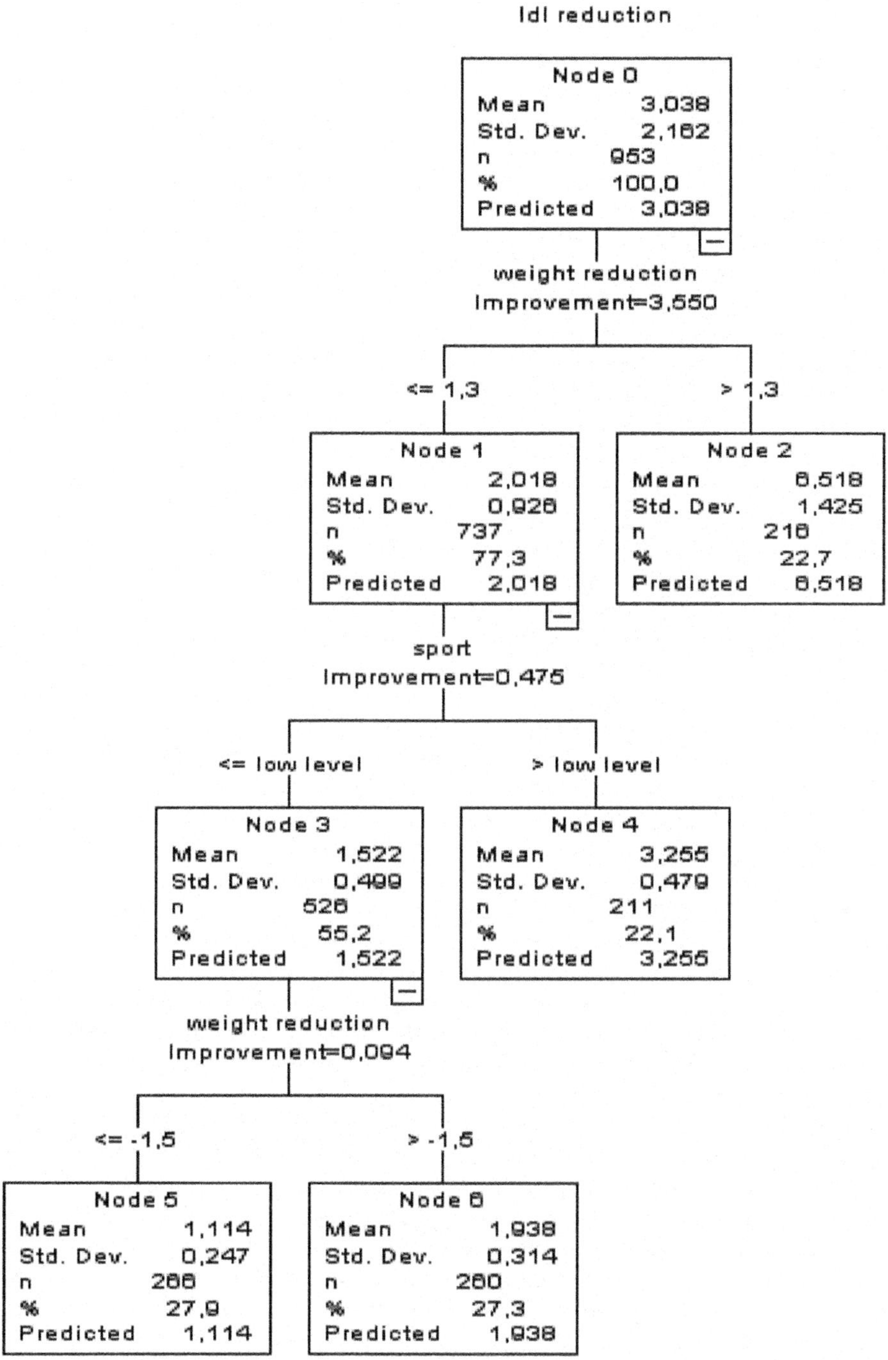
ldl reduction
Node 0
Mean 3,038
Std. Dev. 2,162
n 953
% 100,0
Predicted 3,038
weight reduction
Improvement=3,550
<= 1,3
> 1,3
Node 1
Mean 2,018
Std. Dev. 0,928
n 737
% 77,3
Predicted 2,018
Node 2
Mean 6,518
Std. Dev. 1,425
n 216
% 22,7
Predicted 6,518
sport
Improvement=0,475
<= low level
> low level
Node 3
Mean 1,522
Std. Dev. 0,499
n 526
% 55,2
Predicted 1,522
Node 4
Mean 3,255
Std. Dev. 0,479
n 211
% 22,1
Predicted 3,255
weight reduction
Improvement=0,094
<= -1,5
> -1,5
Node 5
Mean 1,114
Std. Dev. 0,247
n 266
% 27,9
Predicted 1,114
Node 6
Mean 1,938
Std. Dev. 0,314
n 260
% 27,3
Predicted 1,938

The output sheets show the classification (+regression) tree. Only weight reduction and sport significantly contributed to the model, with the overall mean and standard deviation of the dependent variable ldl cholesterol in the parent (root) node. Weight reduction with a cut-off level of 1.3 units is the best predictor of ldl reduction. In the little weight reduction group sport is the best predictor. In the low sport level subgroup again weight reduction is a predictor, but here there is a large difference between weight gain (<−1.5 units) and weight loss (>−1.5 units). Minimizing the output shows the original data file. It now contains two novel variables, the node classification and the predicted value of ldl cholesterol reduction. They are entitled NodeId and PredictedValue. The saved XML (eXtended Markup Language) file will now be used to compute the predicted node classification and value of ldl cholesterol reduction in 5 novel patients with the following characteristics. For convenience the XML file is given in extras.springer.com.

Var 2	Var 3	Var 4	Var 5	Var 6
-,63	1,00	2,00	1,00	,00
2,10	,00	4,00	4,00	1,00
−1,16	1,00	2,00	1,00	1,00
4,22	,00	4,00	1,00	,00
-,59	,00	3,00	4,00	1,00

Var 2 weight_reduction
Var 3 gender
Var 4 sport
Var 5 treatment_level
Var 6 diet

Enter the above data in a new SPSS data file.

Command

Utilities. . . .click Scoring Wizard. . . .click Browse. . . .click Select. . . .Folder: enter the exportdecisiontreecontinuous.xml file. . . .click Select. . . .in Scoring Wizard click Next. . . .mark Node Number. . . .mark Predicted Value. . . .click Next. . . .click Finish.

The above data file now gives individually predicted node classifications and predicted ldl cholesterol reductions as computed by the linear model with the help of the XML file.

Var 2	Var 3	Var 4	Var 5	Var 6	Var 7	Var 8
-,63	1,00	2,00	1,00	,00	6,00	1,94
2,10	,00	4,00	4,00	1,00	2,00	6,52
−1,16	1,00	2,00	1,00	1,00	6,00	1,94
4,22	,00	4,00	1,00	,00	2,00	6,52
−,59	,00	3,00	4,00	1,00	4,00	3,25

Var 2 weight_reduction
Var 3 gender
Var 4 sport
Var 5 treatment_level
Var 6 diet
Var 7 predicted node classification
Var 8 predicted ldl cholesterol reduction

The module decision trees can be readily trained to predict in individual future patients risk of infarction and ldl (low density lipoprotein) cholesterol decrease. Instead of trained XML files for predicting about future patients, also syntax files are possible for the purpose. They perform better, if predictions from multiple, instead of single, future patients are requested.

13.5 Discussion

The effects of risk factors like cholesterol on health risks can be analyzed with chi-squares, if the outcome is binary or with T-tests and analyses of variance, if continuous. However, in order to obtain a more precise information of the magnitude of the effects of various predictors in various subclasses decision trees is a relevant method. Also extended mark-up language files can be constructed for predicting probabilities of a data outcome through regression trees with the help of so-called exhaustive search.

In the current chapter decision trees with continuous outcomes are tested against traditional efficacy analyses with one way anovas. The continuous outcome decision trees provided means and standard deviations of the best fit cut-offs of various subgroups, and, in addition, enabled predictions about future patients through XML files from the experimental data file.

In this chapter the traditional efficacy analysis consisted of one-way analyses of variance, and multiple linear regressions, and the machine learning analyses included continuous decision tree methodologies. The machine learning analyses provided better sensitivity of testing, and were more informative.

13.6 References

To readers requesting more background, theoretical and mathematical information of computations given, several textbooks complementary to the current production and written by the same authors are available:

Statistics applied to clinical studies 5th edition, 2012,
Machine learning in medicine a complete overview, 2015,
SPSS for starters and 2nd levelers 2nd edition, 2015,

Clinical data analysis on a pocket calculator 2nd edition, 2016,
Understanding clinical data analysis from published research, 2016,
Modern meta-analysis, 2017,
Regression analysis in clinical research, 2018,
Modern Bayesian statistics in clinical research, 2018.
The Analysis of Safety Data of Drug Trials, an Update, 2019.

All of them have been edited by Springer Heidelberg Germany.

Chapter 14
Automatic-Data-Mining for Efficacy Analysis

Contents

Abstract In a parallel-group trial of 90 septic patients, the effects of three treatments on laboratory outcomes, and on risks of low blood pressure and those of death were tested, both traditionally, and with the help of machine learning.

Traditional efficacy analysis consisted of

one-way analyses of variance,

3 × 2 crosstabs with 3 × 2 chi-square statistics,

3 dimensional bars of treatment modalities versus outcomes.

Machine learning efficacy analysis consisted of automatic-data-mining methods.

The machine learning methods provided better sensitivity of testing, and were more informative.

Keywords Clinical trials · Traditional efficacy analysis · Machine learning efficacy analysis · Automatic-data-mining methods

T. J. Cleophas, A. H. Zwinderman, *Efficacy Analysis in Clinical Trials an Update*,
https://doi.org/10.1007/978-3-030-19918-0_14

14.1 Introduction

In interventional studies with multiple continuous outcomes, multiple one-way analyses of variances are possible, but these traditional analyses do not account interactions between the outcome variables. SPSS modeler is a work bench for automatic data mining and data modeling. So far it is virtually unused in medicine, and mainly applied by econo-/sociometrists. We will assess whether it can also be used for multiple outcome analysis of clinical data. In data mining the question "is a treatment a predictor of clinical improvement" is assessed by the question "is the outcome, clinical improvement, a predictor of the chance of having had a treatment". This approach may seem incorrect, but is also used with discriminant analysis, and it works fine, because it does not suffer from strong correlations between outcome variables. In this chapter a traditional efficacy analysis will be tested against a machine learning methodology entitled automatic data mining. The traditional efficacy analysis will consist of one-way analyses of variance, 3 × 2 crosstabs with 3 × 2 chi-square statistics, and 3 dimensional bars of treatment modalities versus outcomes.

14.2 Data Example

In this example, 90 patients with sepsis are treated with one of three different treatments. Various outcome values are used as predictors of the output treatment.

asat	alat	ureum	creat	crp	leucos	treat	low-bp	death
5,00	29,00	2,40	79,00	18,00	16,00	1,00	1	0
10,00	30,00	2,10	94,00	15,00	15,00	1,00	1	0
8,00	31,00	2,30	79,00	16,00	14,00	1,00	1	0
6,00	16,00	2,70	80,00	17,00	19,00	1,00	1	0
6,00	16,00	2,20	84,00	18,00	20,00	1,00	1	0
5,00	13,00	2,10	78,00	17,00	21,00	1,00	1	0
10,00	16,00	3,10	85,00	20,00	18,00	1,00	1	0
8,00	28,00	8,00	68,00	15,00	18,00	1,00	1	0
7,00	27,00	7,80	74,00	16,00	17,00	1,00	1	0
6,00	26,00	8,40	69,00	18,00	16,00	1,00	1	0
12,00	22,00	2,70	75,00	14,00	19,00	1,00	1	0
21,00	21,00	3,00	70,00	15,00	20,00	1,00	1	0
10,00	20,00	23,00	74,00	15,00	18,00	1,00	1	0
19,00	19,00	2,10	75,00	16,00	16,00	1,00	1	0
8,00	32,00	2,00	85,00	18,00	19,00	1,00	2	0
20,00	11,00	2,90	63,00	18,00	18,00	1,00	1	0
7,00	30,00	6,80	72,00	17,00	18,00	1,00	1	0
1973,00	846,00	73,80	563,00	18,00	38,00	3,00	2	0
1863,00	757,00	41,70	574,00	15,00	34,00	3,00	2	1
1973,00	646,00	38,90	861,00	16,00	38,00	3,00	2	1

asat = aspartate aminotransferase
alat = alanine aminotransferase
creat = creatinine
crp = c-reactive protein
treat = treatments 1-3
low-bp = low blood pressure (1 no, 2 slight, 3 severe)
death = death (0 no, 1 yes)

Only the first 20 patients are above, the entire data file is in extra.springer.com and is entitled "spssmodeler". SPSS statistical software is used for the traditional efficacy analysis. Start by opening SPSS statistical software in your computer mounted with the software program.

14.3 Traditional Efficacy Analysis

Multiple one-way analyses of variance (ANOVAs) of the treatment modalities on the outcomes will be performed first.

Command

Analyze....Compare Means....One-Way ANOVA....Dependent List: asat.... Factor: treatment....click OK.

In the output sheets is the underneath table.

ANOVA

asat

	Sum of Squares	df	Mean Square	F	Sig.
Between Groups	16351909,50	2	8175954,755	87,538	,000
Within Groups	8125725,480	87	93399,143		
Total	24477634,98	89			

Obviously, the treatment modality is a very significant predictor of the outcome alat. Similarly, five more outcome variables are tested. The output sheets are below.

ANOVA

alat

	Sum of Squares	df	Mean Square	F	Sig.
Between Groups	6268464,905	2	3134232,453	98,028	,000
Within Groups	2781627,595	87	31972,731		
Total	9050092,500	89			

ANOVA

ureum

	Sum of Squares	df	Mean Square	F	Sig.
Between Groups	21015,713	2	10507,856	73,627	,000
Within Groups	12416,428	87	142,718		
Total	33432,141	89			

ANOVA

creatinine

	Sum of Squares	df	Mean Square	F	Sig.
Between Groups	3132958,855	2	1566479,428	83,158	,000
Within Groups	1638847,245	87	18837,325		
Total	4771806,100	89			

ANOVA

c-reactive protein

	Sum of Squares	df	Mean Square	F	Sig.
Between Groups	19003,680	2	9501,840	10,013	,000
Within Groups	82556,320	87	948,923		
Total	101560,000	89			

ANOVA

leucos

	Sum of Squares	df	Mean Square	F	Sig.
Between Groups	3550,300	2	1775,150	62,605	,000
Within Groups	2466,855	87	28,355		
Total	6017,156	89			

Obviously, all of the other laboratory outcomes were also significantly predicted by the treatment modalities.

The effect of treatment on death was assessed with a 3 × 2 crosstab and a 3 × 2 chi-square test.

Command

Analyze....Descriptives....Crosstab....Row(s): treatment....Column: death.... Statistics: mark Chi-square....click Continue....click OK.

treatment * death Crosstabulation

Count

		death		Total
		no	yes	
treatment	1,00	33	2	35
	2,00	12	24	36
	3,00	3	16	19
Total		48	42	90

Chi-Square Tests

	Value	df	Asymp. Sig. (2-sided)
Pearson Chi-Square	40,130[a]	2	,000
Likelihood Ratio	46,631	2	,000
N of Valid Cases	90		

a. 0 cells (,0%) have expected count less than 5. The minimum expected count is 8,87.

The above table in the output shows a very significant effect on death of the treatment modalities. A 3-D chart is helpful for visualizing purpose.

Command

click Graphs....Legacy Dialogs....3-D Bar....Groups of Cases....Rows: Treatment....Columns: death....click OK.

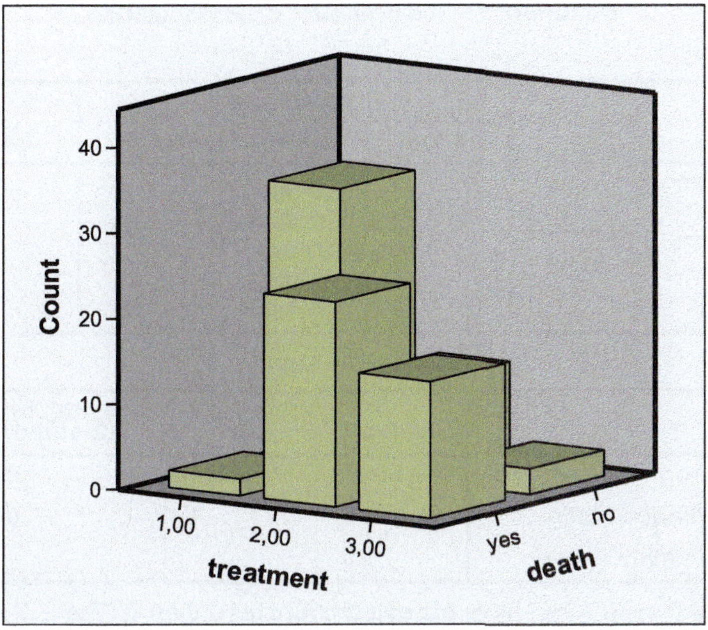

Conclusions from the above analyses are given.

1. All of the lab predictors were very significant predictors of death in the one-way ANOVAs (analyses of variance).
2. The treatments were assessed with a crosstab (3 × 2 interaction matrix), and were also a very significant predictor of death.
3. In order to understand how the treatments benefited results, a 3 dimensional bar chart was drawn. There were many survivors in the treatment 1, and few survivors in the treatment 2 and 3 patients, consistent with the result from the above crosstab.

We were also interested in the effects of treatment on blood pressures.
Again a 3 × 2 crosstab was applied. Command.

Command

click Graphs....Legacy Dialogs....3-D Bar....Groups of Cases....Rows: Treatment....Columns: blood pressure....click OK.

treatment * blood pressure Crosstabulation

Count

		blood pressure			Total
		normal	low	very low	
treatment	1,00	29	4	2	35
	2,00	3	13	20	36
	3,00	0	11	8	19
Total		32	28	30	90

Chi-Square Tests

	Value	df	Asymp. Sig. (2-sided)
Pearson Chi-Square	59,094[a]	4	,000
Likelihood Ratio	67,007	4	,000
N of Valid Cases	90		

a. 0 cells (,0%) have expected count less than 5. The minimum expected count is 5,91.

The above tables were in the output, and showed a very significant effect of treatment on blood pressures. A 3-D chart is helpful for visualizing purpose.

Command

click Graphs….Legacy Dialogs….3-D Bar….Groups of Cases….Rows: Treatment….Columns: death….click OK.

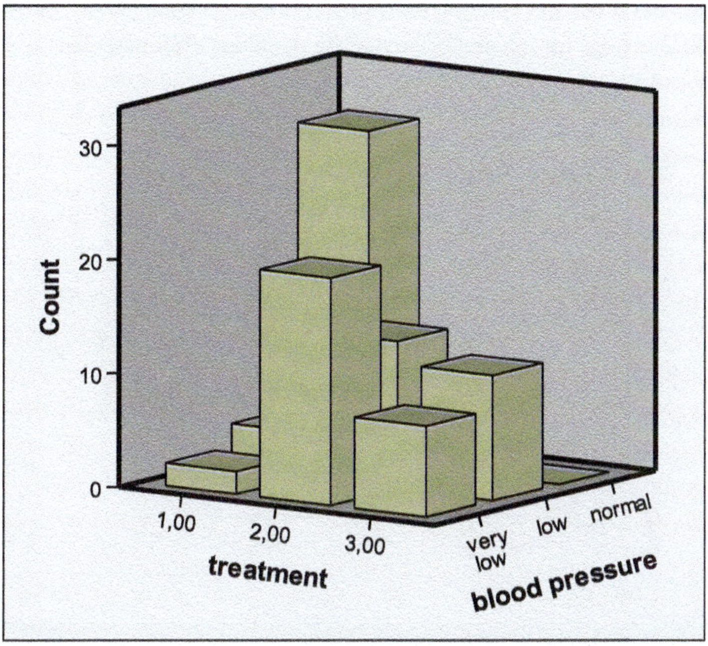

The above graph is in the output, and shows many treatment 1 patients with normal blood pressure, and many treatments 2 and 3 with low blood pressures. In order to find support, whether treatment modality is not only a direct predictor of survival, but also is a predictor of clinical improvement as measured with multiple lab levels, an automatic data mining procedure was performed with the help of SPSS Modeler, a work bench for automatic data mining and data modeling.

14.4 Automatic-Data-Mining for Efficacy Analysis

SPSS modeler is a work bench for automatic data mining, and data modeling. So far it is virtually unused in medicine, and mainly applied by econo-/sociometrists. We will assess, whether it can also be used for multiple outcome analysis of clinical data.

The above data example was used once again. Patients with sepsis had been given one of three treatments. Various outcome variables had been used to assess which one of the treatments performs best.

In data mining the question "is a treatment a predictor of clinical improvement" is assessed by the question "is the outcome, clinical improvement, a predictor of the chance of having had a treatment". This approach may seem incorrect, but is also used with discriminant analysis, and works fine, because it does not suffer from strong correlations between outcome variables. In this example, 90 patients with sepsis had been treated with one of three different treatments. Various outcome values are used as predictors of the output treatment.

The data file is in extra.springer.com and is entitled "spssmodeler". SPSS modeler version 14.2 is used for the analysis. Start by opening SPSS modeler.

14.4.1 Step 1 Open SPSS Modeler

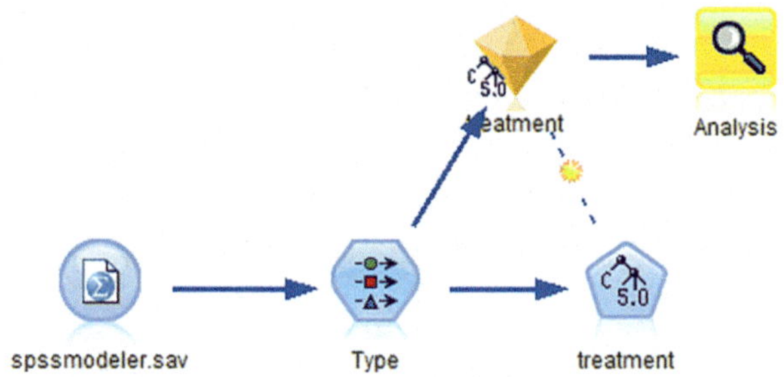

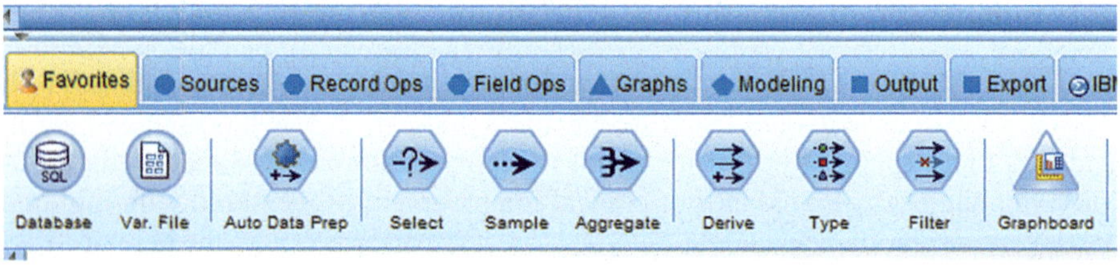

In the palettes at the bottom of the screen full of nodes, look and find the **Statistics File node**, and drag it to the canvas. Double-click on it. . . .Import file: browse and enter the file "spssmodeler.sav". . . .click OK. . . .in the palette find **Distribution node** and drag to canvas. . . .right-click on the Statistics File node. . . .a Connect symbol comes up. . . .click on the Distribution node. . . .an arrow is displayed. . . . double-click on the Distribution Node. . . .after a second or two the underneath graph with information from the Distribution node is observed.

14.4.2 Step 2 the Distribution Node

Value	Proportion	%	Count
1.00		38.89	35
2.00		40.0	36
3.00		21.11	19

It gives the frequency distribution of the three treatments in the 90 patient data file. All of the treatments are substantially present.

Next remove the Distribution node by clicking on it and press delete on the key board of your computer. Continue by dragging the Data audit node to the canvas.... perform the connecting manoeuvres as above....double-click it again.

14.4.3 Step 3 the Data Audit Node

Field	Graph	Measurement	Min	Max	Mean	Std. Dev	Skewness	Unique	Valid
asat		Continuous	5.000	2000.000	360.789	524.433	2.004	--	90
alat		Continuous	11.000	976.000	280.833	318.883	1.036	--	90
ureum		Continuous	2.000	83.000	20.310	19.381	1.338	--	90
creatinine		Continuous	59.000	861.000	272.767	231.551	0.967	--	90
creactiveprotein		Continuous	14.000	131.000	41.667	33.781	1.360	--	90
leucos		Continuous	14.000	42.000	26.822	8.222	0.151	--	90
treatment		Nominal	1.000	3.000	--	--	--	3	90
lowbloodpress...		Nominal	--	--	--	--	--	3	90
death		Nominal	--	--	--	--	--	2	90

The Data audit will be edited. Select "treatment" as target field (field is variable here)....click Run. The information from this node is now given in the form of a Data audit plot, showing that due to the treatment low values are frequently more often observed than the high values. Particularly, the treatments 1 and 2 (light blue and red) are often associated with low values, these are probably the best treatments. Next remove the Data audit node by clicking on it and press delete on the key board of your computer. Continue by dragging the Plot node to the canvas. . . .perform the connecting manoeuvres as above. . . .double-click it again.

14.4.4 Step 4 the Plot Node

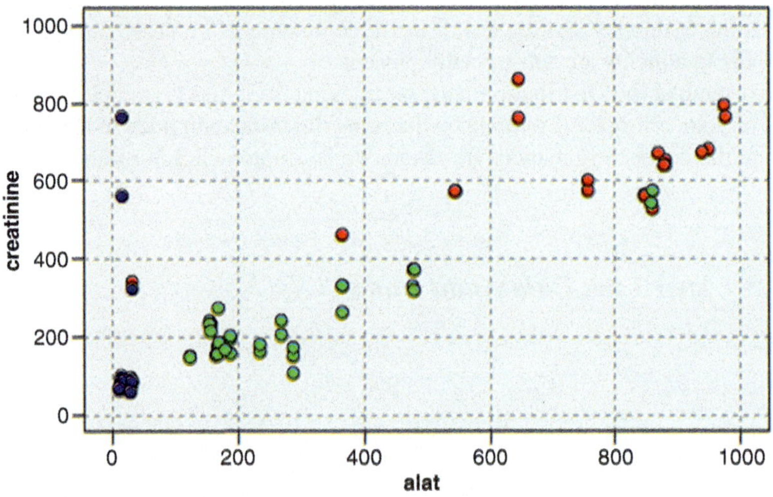

The Plot node will be edited. On the Plot tab select creatinine as y-variable and alat as x-variable, and treatment in the Overlay field at Color. . . .click Run. The information from this node is now given in the form of a scatter plot of patients. This scatter plot of alat versus creatinine values shows that the three treatments are somewhat separately clustered. Treatment 1 (blue) in the left lower part, 2 (green) in the middle, and 3 in the right upper part. Low values means adequate effect of treatment. So treatment 1 (and also some patients with treatment 2) again perform pretty well. Next remove the Plot node by clicking on it and press delete on the key board of your computer. Continue by dragging the Web node to the canvas. . . . perform the connecting manoeuvres as above. . . .double-click it again.

14.4.5 Step 5 the Web Node

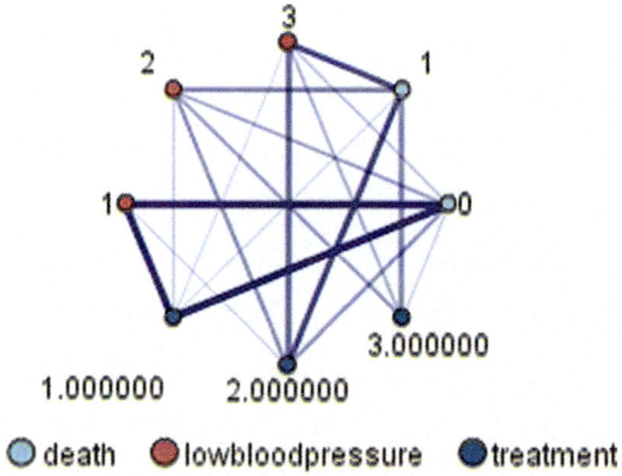

The Web node will be edited. In the Web note dialog box click Select All. . . .click Run. The web graph that comes up, shows that treatment 1 (indicated here as 1.000000) is strongly associated with no death and no low blood pressure (thick line), which is very good. However, the treatments 2 (2.000000) and 3 (3.000000) are strongly associated with death and treatment 2 (2.000000) is also associated with the severest form of low blood pressure. Next remove the Web node by clicking on it and press delete on the key board of your computer. Continue by dragging both the Type and C5.0 nodes to the canvas. . . .perform the connecting manoeuvres respectively as indicated in the first graph of this chapter. . . .double-click it again. . . .a gold nugget is placed as shown above. . . .click the gold nugget.

14.4.6 Step 6 the Type and c5.0 Nodes

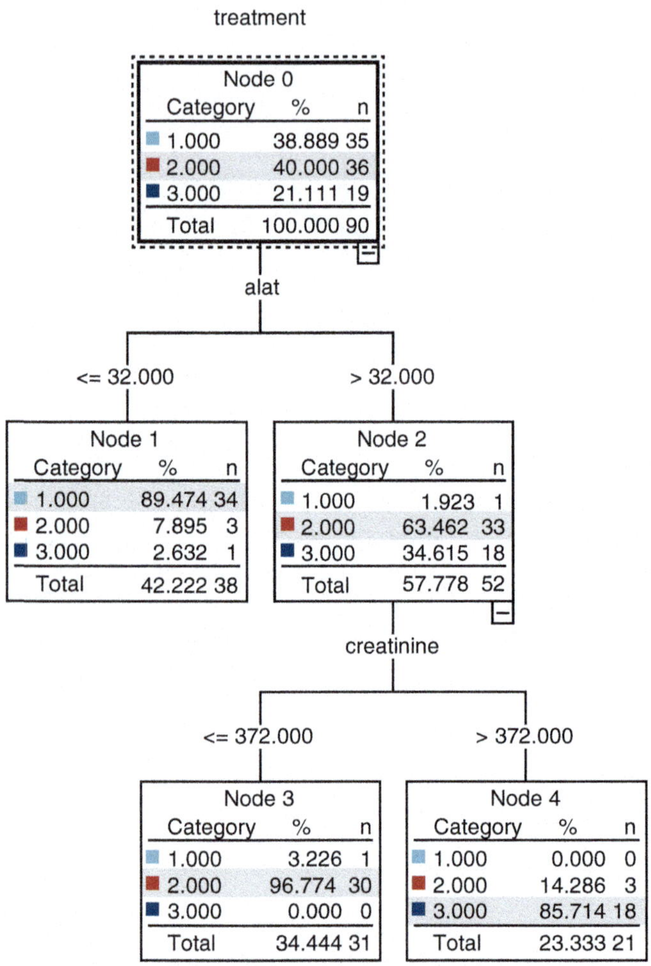

The output sheets give various interactive graphs and tables. One of them is the above C5.0 decision tree. C5.0 decision trees are an improved version of the traditional Quinlan decision trees with less, but more-relevant information.

The C5.0 classifier underscores the previous findings. The variable alat is the best classifier of the treatments with alat < 32 over 89% of the patients having had treatment 1, and with alat > 32 over 63 % of the patients having had treatment 2. Furthermore, in the high alat class patients with a creatinine over 372 around 86 % has treatment 3. And so all in all, the treatment 1 would seem the best treatment and treatment 3 the worst one.

14.4.7 Step 7 the Output Node

Results for output field treatment

Comparing $C-treatment with treatment

Correct	82	91,11%
Wrong	8	8,89%
Total	90	

In order to assess the accuracy of the C5.0 classifier output, an Output node is attached to the gold nugget. Find Output node and drag it to the canvas. . . .perform connecting manoeuvres with the gold nugget. . . .double-click the Output node again. . . .click Run. The output sheet shows an accuracy (true positives and true negatives) of 91,11%, which is pretty good.

14.5 Discussion

In interventional studies with multiple continuous outcomes, one-way analyses of variances are possible for traditional efficacy analyses, but interactions between the outcome variables are not accounted. SPSS modeler is a work bench for automatic data mining and data modeling. So far, it is virtually unused in medicine, and mainly applied by econo-/sociometrists. We assessed, whether it can also be used for multiple outcome analysis of clinical data. In data mining, the question "is a treatment a predictor of clinical improvement" is often assessed by the question ""is the outcome, clinical improvement, a predictor of the chance of having had a treatment". This approach may seem incorrect, but is also used in discriminant analysis, and works fine, because it does not suffer from strong correlations between the outcome variables.

SPSS modeler can be adequately used for multiple outcomes analysis of clinical data. Finding the most appropriate treatment for a disease might be one of the goals of this kind of research. SPSS modeler is a software program entirely distinct from SPSS statistical software, though it uses most if not all of the calculus methods of it. It is a standard software package particularly used by market analysts, but as shown, can perfectly well be applied for the purpose in medical research.

In this chapter the traditional efficacy analysis consisted of one-way analyses of variance, 3 × 2 crosstabs with 3 × 2 chi-square statistics, and 3 dimensional bars of treatment modalities versus outcomes, and the machine learning analyses included automatic data mining methodologies. The machine learning analyses provided better sensitivity of testing, and were more informative.

14.6 References

To readers requesting more background, theoretical and mathematical information of computations given, several textbooks complementary to the current production and written by the same authors are available:

Statistics applied to clinical studies 5th edition, 2012,
Machine learning in medicine a complete overview, 2015,
SPSS for starters and 2nd levelers 2nd edition, 2015,
Clinical data analysis on a pocket calculator 2nd edition, 2016,
Understanding clinical data analysis from published research, 2016,
Modern meta-analysis, 2017,
Regression analysis in clinical research, 2018,
Modern Bayesian statistics in clinical research, 2018.
The Analysis of Safety Data of Drug Trials, an Update, 2019.

All of them have been edited by Springer Heidelberg Germany.

Chapter 15
Support-Vector-Machines for Efficacy Analysis

Contents

Abstract In a random 200 septic patient sample, the effect of laboratory values on the risk of death was tested, both traditionally, and with help of machine learning.

Traditional efficacy analysis was composed of
discretization of continuous predictors,
crosstabs with chi-square statistics,
multiple binary logistic regressions.

Machine learning efficacy analysis was composed of support-vector-machine methods.

The machine learning methods provided better sensitivity of testing, and were more informative.

Keywords Clinical trials · Traditional efficacy analysis · Machine learning efficacy analysis · Support-vector-machines methods

15.1 Introduction

Laboratory values are sometimes used as surrogate factors for making predictions about health outcomes. For example, hepatic, renal, inflammatory markers are used for the purpose. If the health outcomes are discrete like morbidity or mortality, then

T. J. Cleophas, A. H. Zwinderman, *Efficacy Analysis in Clinical Trials an Update*,
https://doi.org/10.1007/978-3-030-19918-0_15

transformation of continuous laboratory values into discrete ones enables to perform traditional efficacy analyses using crosstabs and chi-squares tests. As an alternative cluster analyses are possible. Cluster analyses are generally computationally intensive, and, with big data, computations may even take weeks or months, because the distance between each datum to all other data is measured. Support vector machines is a clever method for cluster identification. Unlike methods like neural networks, it does not use all observations, but only the observations that are very close to the separation lines of two clusters. Rather than all observations, the difficult ones, the ones lying close to the separation line are applied. The basic aim of support vector machines is to construct the best fit separation line (or with three dimensional data separation plane), and to identify the separating cases and controls as good as possible. The method is particularly suitable for imperfect nonlinear data. Discriminant analysis, classification trees, and neural networks are alternative methods for the purpose, but support vector machines are generally more stable and sensitive, although heuristic studies to indicate, when they perform better, are missing. Support vector machines are also used in automatic modeling, that computes ensembled results of multiple best fit models. This chapter uses the Konstanz information miner (Knime), a free data mining software package developed at the University of Konstanz for the machine learning method called support vector machines. The traditional efficacy analysis in this chapter will consist of discretized continuous predictors, crosstabs with chi-square statistics, and multiple binary logistic regressions.

15.2 Data Example

Is support vector machines adequate to classify cases and controls in a sample of patients admitted because of sepsis? Two hundred patients were admitted because of sepsis. The laboratory values and the outcome death or alive were registered. We wish to use support vector machines to predict from the laboratory values the outcome, death or alive, including information on the error rates. The data of the first 12 patients are underneath. The entire data file is in extras.springer.com, and is entitled “ensembledmodelbinary”. Konstanz information miner (Knime) does not use SPSS files, and, so, the file has to be transformed into a csv excel file (click Save As….then in “Save as” type: replace SPSS Statistics(∗sav) with SPSS Statistics (∗csv). For convenience the csv file is in extras.springer.com and is entitled “svm” (var = variable).

Death 1= yes	Ggt	asat	alat	bili	ureum	creat	c-clear	esr	crp	leucos
var1	**var2**	**var3**	**var4**	**var5**	**var6**	**var7**	**var8**	**var9**	**Var10**	**var11**
0	20	23	34	2	3,4	89	-111	2	2	5
0	14	21	33	3	2	67	-112	7	3	6
0	30	35	32	4	5,6	58	-116	8	4	4
0	35	34	40	4	6	76	-110	6	5	7
0	23	33	22	4	6,1	95	-120	9	6	6
0	26	31	24	3	5,4	78	-132	8	4	8
0	15	29	26	2	5,3	47	-120	12	5	5
0	13	26	24	1	6,3	65	-132	13	6	6
0	26	27	27	4	6	97	-112	14	6	7
0	34	25	13	3	4	67	-125	15	7	6
0	32	26	24	3	3,6	58	-110	13	8	6
0	21	13	15	3	3,6	69	-102	12	2	4

Var 1 death 1 = yes
Var 2 gammagt (Var = variable) (U/l)
Var 3 asat (U/l)
Var 4 alat (U/l)
Var 5 bili (mumol/l)
Var 6 ureum (mmol/l)
Var 7 creatinine (mumol/l)
Var 8 creatinine clearance (ml/min)
Var 9 esr (erythrocyte sedimentation rate) (mm)
Var 10 c-reactive protein (mg/l)
Var 11 leucos ($x10^9$ /l)

15.3 Traditional Efficacy Analysis

Traditional efficacy analysis consists of t-tests for continuous outcomes and chi-square tests for discrete outcomes. In Sect. 1.12, Chap. 1, the use of regression analyses for efficacy analyses is discussed, and in Sect. 1.13 the use of clinical trials for the assessment of causal health effects of factors other than medicines is discussed. For example, effects of interventions like angioplasties, surgeries, renal transplants etc. Many more factors can be tested in clinical trials, for example,

age factors
psychological factors
social factors
physical factors
economical factors,
and, any factor with a supposedly causal effect on health or sickness.

In the current chapter, start by opening the data file in your computer with SPSS statistical software installed.

Command

click Analyze. . . .Descriptive Statistics. . . .Descriptives. . . .Variable(s). . . .enter Var 00001 to 00011. . . .click OK.

The means and standard deviations are given in the output.

Descriptive Statistics

	N	Minimum	Maximum	Mean	Std. Deviation
gammagt	200	2,00	2300,00	200,4950	349,59912
asat	200	3,00	1980,00	194,3950	335,60735
alat	200	2,00	1500,00	190,5400	308,25185
bili	200	1,00	400,00	62,0900	94,28793
ureum	200	2,00	98,00	15,2525	19,02840
creatinine	200	47,00	865,00	192,8100	190,15517
creatinine clearance	200	-132,00	-4,00	-80,1200	41,94188
esr	200	2,00	180,00	38,9200	39,69170
c-reactive protein	200	2,00	243,00	23,2400	35,37839
leucos	200	2,00	30,00	12,0450	7,75912
Valid N (listwise)	200				

We will apply the means from the above table for cut-offs for the purpose of discretization of the continuous variables.

Command

Transform. . . .Compute Variable. . . .Target Variable: write the term ggt. . . .Numeric Expression: enter gammagt. . . .click ">" from the underneath blue calculator. . . .then click "200". . . .click OK.

In the data screen now a novel variable entitled ggt is observed. We will test the significance of difference between the two groups of predictors on numbers of deaths.

		death no	death yes
Group 1	ggt < 200	a	b
Group 2	ggt > 200	c	d

For that purpose a chi-square test of the above 2 × 2 crosstab will be performed. Command.

Command

Analyze. . . .Descriptives. . . .Crosstabs. . . .Rows: enter ggt. . . .Column (s). . . .click Statistics. . . .mark chi-square. . . .click Continue. . . .click OK.

The tables below are in the output sheets.

ggt * death Crosstabulation

Count

		death		Total
		,00	1,00	
ggt	,00	107	41	148
	1,00	0	52	52
Total		107	93	200

Chi-Square Tests

	Value	df	Asymp. Sig. (2-sided)	Exact Sig. (2-sided)	Exact Sig. (1-sided)
Pearson Chi-Square	80,849[a]	1	,000		
Continuity Correction[b]	77,969	1	,000		
Likelihood Ratio	101,602	1	,000		
Fisher's Exact Test				,000	,000
Linear-by-Linear Association	80,444	1	,000		
N of Valid Cases	200				

a. 0 cells (,0%) have expected count less than 5. The minimum expected count is 24,18.
b. Computed only for a 2x2 table

No deaths were in the group with ggt < 200. Although the chi-square is flawed with cells smaller than 5 subjects, the p-values of 0.000 suggests that ggt is a very strong surrogate factor of death. In the same way, all of the surrogate factors were applied for testing.

All of the p-values were < 0.000, and the chi-square values were very high.

laboratory values	chi-square values
gamma gt	80.8
asat	88.0
alat	83.0
bili	99.6
ureum	85.8
creatinine	77.9
creatinine clearance	137.7
esr	102
c-reactive protein	90.3
leucos	148.4

The best chi-squares were those from the leucocyte counts and the creatinine clearances. The analyses were univariate, and, so, confoundings and interactions of the predictors on the outcome were not taken into account.

A multiple logistic regression with all of the undiscretized predictors was performed.

Command

Analyze. . . .Regression. . . .Binary Logistic. . . .Dependent: enter death. . . .Covariate (s): enter: all of the original predictors. . . .click OK.

In the output only 3 predictors remained independent: Var 00005 (bili), 00010 (c-reactive protein), 00011 (leucos).

Variables in the Equation

		B	S.E.	Wald	df	Sig.	Exp(B)
Step 1[a]	VAR00002	,020	,019	1,141	1	,285	1,020
	VAR00003	,003	,017	,034	1	,854	1,003
	VAR00004	,001	,015	,002	1	,965	1,001
	VAR00005	,038	,017	5,237	1	,022	1,039
	VAR00006	-,172	,112	2,350	1	,125	,842
	VAR00007	,001	,008	,016	1	,901	1,001
	VAR00008	-,036	,034	1,147	1	,284	,964
	VAR00009	-,021	,049	,187	1	,665	,979
	VAR00010	-,068	,033	4,270	1	,039	,934
	VAR00011	1,236	,395	9,781	1	,002	3,442
	Constant	-17,739	6,609	7,205	1	,007	,000

a. Variable(s) entered on step 1: VAR00002, VAR00003, VAR00004, VAR00005, VAR00006, VAR00007, VAR00008, VAR00009, VAR00010, VAR00011.

A multiple logistic regression with all of the discretized predictors was, subsequently, performed.

Command

Analyze....Regression....Binary Logistic....Dependent: enter death....Covariate (s): enter: all of the discretized predictors....click OK.

In the output now only 2 predictors remained independent: creatinine clearance and leucocyte count. But they were significant at better levels of significance than the predictors of the undiscretized analysis were.

Variables in the Equation

		B	S.E.	Wald	df	Sig.	Exp(B)
Step 1[a]	ggt	90,453	6008,584	,000	1	,988	1,919E39
	asat	-10,832	1361,181	,000	1	,994	,000
	alat	57,649	4587,495	,000	1	,990	1,088E25
	bili	1,198	2,654	,204	1	,652	3,313
	ureum	33,467	2837,424	,000	1	,991	3,425E14
	creatinine	-57,013	4142,290	,000	1	,989	,000
	creatinineclearance	-3,729	,823	20,547	1	,000	,024
	esr	33,300	2697,568	,000	1	,990	2,897E14
	creactp	-12,008	1350,962	,000	1	,993	,000
	leuco	3,344	1,093	9,350	1	,002	28,319
	Constant	,121	,610	,040	1	,842	1,129

a. Variable(s) entered on step 1: ggt, asat, alat, bili, ureum, creatinine, creatinineclearance, esr, creactp, leuco.

The efficacy analysis underscored the usefulness of laboratory values as surrogates for predicting mortality in patients with sepsis. However, the analyses were largely univariate, and interactions between the predictors on the outcome were not taken into account. Multiple logistic regressions with undiscretized predictors were exploratory rather than confirmative analyses.

15.4 Support-Vector-Machines for Efficacy Analysis

As an alternative, cluster analyses may provide helpful information so far missing in the above traditional analysis. Support vector machines is a clever method for cluster identification. Unlike machine learning methods like neural networks, it does not use all data, but only the observations that are very close to the separation lines. The basic aim of support vector machines is to construct the best fit separation line (or with three dimensional data separation plane), as well as separating cases and controls as good as possible. The method is particularly suitable for imperfect nonlinear data. Discriminant analysis, classification trees, and neural networks are alternative methods for the purpose, but support vector machines are generally more stable and sensitive, although heuristic studies to indicate, when they perform better are missing. In Google enter the term "knime". Click Download and follow instructions. After completing the pretty easy download procedure, open the knime workbench by clicking the knime welcome screen. The center of the screen displays the workflow editor like the canvas in SPSS modeler. It is empty, and can be used to build a stream of nodes, called workflow in knime. The node repository is in the left lower angle of the screen, and the nodes can be dragged to the workflow editor simply by left-clicking. The nodes are computer tools for data analysis like visualization and statistical processes. Node description is in the right upper angle of the screen. Before the nodes can be used they have to be connected with the file reader and with one another by arrows drawn again simply by left clicking the small triangles attached to the nodes. Right clicking on the file reader enables to configure from your computer a requested data file.

The knime (Konstanz information miner) has already been used for many analyses in this edition. It will be used again for the analysis of the current data example. First, a workflow will be built, and the final result is shown in the underneath figure

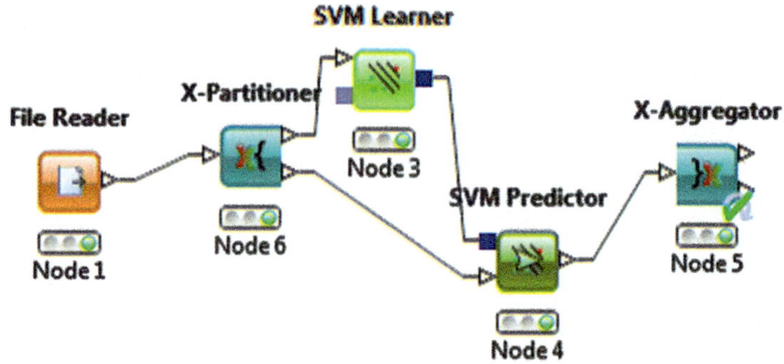

15.4.1 File Reader Node

In the node repository find the node File Reader. Drag the node to the workflow editor by left clicking. . . .click Browse. . . .and download from extras.springer.com the csv type Excel file entitled "svm". You are set for analysis now. By left clicking the node the file is displayed. The File Reader has chosen Var 0006 (ureum) as S variable (dependent). However, we wish to replace it with Var 0001 (death yes = 1). . . .click the column header of Var 0006. . . .mark "Don't include column in output". . . .click OK. . . .in the column header of Var 0001 leave unmarked "Don't include column in output". . . .click OK.

The outcome variable is now rightly the Var 0001 and is indicated with S, the Var 0006 has obtained the term "SKIP"between brackets.

15.4.2 *The Nodes X-Partitioner, SVM Learner, SVM Predictor, X-Aggregator*

Find the above nodes in the node repository and drag them to the workflow editor and connect them with one another according to the above figure. Configurate and execute all them by right clicking the nodes and the texts "Configurate" and "Execute". The red lights under the nodes get, subsequently, yellow and, then, green. The miner has accomplished its task.

15.4.3 *Error Rates*

Right click the X-Aggregator node once more, and then right click Error rates. The underneath table is shown. The svm (support vector machine) model is used to make predictions about death or not from the other variables of your file. Nine random samples of 25 patients are shown. The error rates are pretty small, and vary from 0 to 12.5%. We should add that other measures of uncertainty like sensitivity or specificity are not provided by knime.

Error rates - 0:5 - X-Aggregator

File

Table "default" - Rows: 10 | Spec - Columns: 3 | Properties | Flow Variables

Row ID	D Error in %	I Size of ...	I Error C...
fold 0	4	25	1
fold 1	4	25	1
fold 2	4.167	24	1
fold 3	12	25	3
fold 4	4.167	24	1
fold 5	8	25	2
fold 6	12	25	3
fold 7	0	24	0
fold 8	8	25	2
fold 9	12.5	24	3

15.4.4 *Prediction Table*

Right click the x-aggregator node once more, and then right click Prediction Table. The underneath table is shown. The svm model is used to make predictions about death or not from the other variables of your file.

The left column gives the outcome values (death yes = 1), the right one gives the predicted values. It can be observed that the two results very well match one another.

Prediction table - 0:5 - X-Aggregator

File

Table "default" - Rows: 246 | Spec - Columns: 11 | Properties | Flow Variables

Row ID	S ï»¿VAR...	I VAROO...	I VAROO...	I VAROO...	I VAROO...	I VAROO...	I VAROO...	I VAROO...	I VAROO...	I VAROO...	S Predicti...
Row4	0	23	33	22	4	95	-120	9	6	6	0
Row6	0	15	29	26	2	47	-120	12	5	5	0
Row9	0	34	25	13	3	67	-125	15	7	6	0
Row14	0	19	16	9	4	80	-113	8	4	7	0
Row18	0	24	24	27	4	84	-120	15	6	6	0
Row36	0	19	236	15	2	78	-113	7	6	6	0
Row42	0	27	17	27	4	98	-101	14	4	3	0
Row47	0	15	17	15	2	89	-112	13	9	6	0
Row62	0	16	14	19	4	67	-102	14	7	2	0
Row64	0	14	14	27	2	76	-109	18	5	5	0
Row66	0	16	27	29	3	77	-102	14	4	6	0
Row67	0	24	25	24	2	69	-110	16	5	7	0
Row68	0	21	29	25	4	78	-112	15	7	4	0
Row73	0	21	15	13	2	92	-120	17	7	4	0
Row114	1	900	759	856	287	532	-8	109	103	23	1
Row144	1	376	459	389	135	267	-29	97	33	20	1
Row151	1	169	154	267	75	244	-50	42	21	15	1
Row155	1	175	250	276	95	231	-41	36	28	15	1
Row170	1	276	230	156	79	235	-54	34	23	15	1
Row181	1	75	84	145	39	137	-66	28	18	14	1

15.5 Discussion

The basic aim of support vector machines is to construct the best fit separation line (or with three dimensional data separation plane), separating cases and controls as good as possible. This chapter uses the Konstanz information miner, a free data mining software package developed at the University of Konstanz. The example shows that support vector machines is adequate to predict the presence of a disease or not in a cohort of patients at risk of a disease.

The traditional efficacy analysis in this chapter underscored the usefulness of laboratory values as surrogates for predicting mortality in patients with sepsis. However, the analyses were largely univariate, and confoundings and interactions of the predictors on the outcome were not taken into account. Multiple logistic regressions with undiscretized predictors were exploratory rather than confirmative analyses. The machine learning method here applied showed that the support vector clusters accurately predicted measured outcomes.

In this chapter the traditional efficacy analysis consisted of discretized continuous predictors, and crosstabs with chi-square statistics multiple binary logistic regressions, and the machine learning analyses included support vector machines. The machine learning analyses provided better sensitivity of testing, and were more informative.

15.6 References

To readers requesting more background, theoretical and mathematical information of computations given, several textbooks complementary to the current production and written by the same authors are available:

Statistics applied to clinical studies 5th edition, 2012,
Machine learning in medicine a complete overview, 2015,
SPSS for starters and 2nd levelers 2nd edition, 2015,
Clinical data analysis on a pocket calculator 2nd edition, 2016,
Understanding clinical data analysis from published research, 2016,
Modern meta-analysis, 2017,
Regression analysis in clinical research, 2018,
Modern Bayesian statistics in clinical research, 2018.
The Analysis of Safety Data of Drug Trials, an Update, 2019.

All of them have been edited by Springer Heidelberg Germany.

Chapter 16
Neural-Networks for Efficacy Analysis

Contents

Abstract In a 250 patient self-controlled study of drug efficacy scores, measured as differences from baseline, the effect of highly expressed gene polymorphisms on drug efficacy scores was tested, both traditionally and with the help of machine learning.

Traditional efficacy analysis consisted of
discretization of continuous predictors,
3 × 2 crosstabs with 3 × 2 chi-square statistics.
Machine learning efficacy analysis was composed of neural-network methods.
The machine learning methods provided better sensitivity of testing, and were more informative.

Keywords Clinical trials · Traditional efficacy analysis · Machine learning efficacy analysis · Neural-network methods

16.1 Introduction

The effect of discrete predictors like lifestyle levels on health levels can be analyzed with traditional crosstabs and chi-square tests. To better account for nonlinear relationships neural networks are more appropriate than traditional testing. Radial basis functions (RBFs), as applied in radial basis neural networks, is equivalent to Gaussian kernel regression. It may, better than multilayer perceptron neural network, predict medical data, because it uses a Gaussian activation function, but it is rarely

T. J. Cleophas, A. H. Zwinderman, *Efficacy Analysis in Clinical Trials an Update*,
https://doi.org/10.1007/978-3-030-19918-0_16

used. This chapter is to test its performance in clinical trials against that of traditional efficacy analytics. Quality of life (qol) is multidimensional, and factors like age, gender, being married, and lifestyle may be independent determinants, although maybe rather in a nonlinear and categorical than linear way. Can a radial basis neural network be applied to accurately predict the effect of the above factors on qol. In this chapter the traditional efficacy analysis will be tested against a machine learning method called radial basis neural networks, here used for efficacy analysis. The traditional efficacy analysis will consist of discretized continuous predictors, and 3×2 crosstabs with 3×2 chi-square statistics.

16.2 Data Example

In a 445 patient study the effects of age, gender, being married, and lifestyle levels on quality of life (qol) levels were assessed. The underneath table shows the data of the first 12 patients

qol	age	gender	married	lifestyle
2	55	1	0	0
2	32	1	1	1
1	27	1	1	0
3	77	0	1	0
1	34	1	1	0
1	35	1	0	1
2	57	1	1	1
2	57	1	1	1
1	35	0	0	0
2	42	1	1	0
3	30	0	1	0
1	34	0	1	1

The entire data file is in extras.springer.com, and is entitled "radialbasisneuralnetwork".

16.3 Traditional Efficacy Analysis

the traditional efficacy analysis consisted of 3×2 crosstabs with 3×2 chi-square tests, with predictors as row variable, and qol as column variable. The analysis may be adequate for identifying the most important predictors of the outcome categories of qol, but with nonlinear relationships better sensitivity of testing may be obtained with multilayer neural networks propagating a received signal beyond some threshold forward to a next layer. Radial basis neural networks are used for the purpose.

Except for age all of the predictor variables were discrete. Start by opening the data file entitled "radialbasisneuralnetwork", in your computer mounted with SPSS statistical software. First, we will transform the continuous variable age in a discrete variable.

Command

Analyze....Descriptives....Descriptive Statistics....Variables: enter age.... click OK.

The table underneath given in the output shows, that the mean age is 50 years. This will be used as cut-off for discretization.

Descriptive Statistics

	N	Minimum	Maximum	Mean	Std. Deviation
age	445	20	77	49,72	14,304
Valid N (listwise)	445				

In the data screen view a novel, binary, variable is observed called agelevel.

qol	age	gender	married	lifestyle	agelevel
2	55	1	0	0	1,00
2	32	1	1	1	,00
1	27	1	1	0	,00
3	77	0	1	0	1,00
1	34	1	1	0	,00
1	35	1	0	1	,00
2	57	1	1	1	1,00
2	57	1	1	1	1,00
1	35	0	0	0	,00
2	42	1	1	0	,00
3	30	0	1	0	,00
1	34	0	1	1	,00

We will now use this novel variable for making predictions about the effect of age on qol, using from the descriptives menu the crosstab command.

Command

Analyze....Descriptives....Crosstabs....Row(s): agelevel....Column: qol.... click OK.

Output sheets are below.

qol * agelevel Crosstabulation

Count

		agelevel		Total
		,00	1,00	
qol	low	118	3	121
	medium	82	90	172
	high	5	147	152
Total		205	240	445

Chi-Square Tests

	Value	df	Asymp. Sig. (2-sided)
Pearson Chi-Square	241,066[a]	2	,000
Likelihood Ratio	303,989	2	,000
Linear-by-Linear Association	240,210	1	,000
N of Valid Cases	445		

a. 0 cells (,0%) have expected count less than 5. The minimum expected count is 55,74.

Obviously, age level was a very significant predictor of qol. Subsequently, the other predictors were tested similarly.

qol * gender Crosstabulation

Count

		gender		Total
		Male	Female	
qol	low	60	61	121
	medium	89	83	172
	high	73	79	152
Total		222	223	445

Chi-Square Tests

	Value	df	Asymp. Sig. (2-sided)
Pearson Chi-Square	,452[a]	2	,798
Likelihood Ratio	,452	2	,798
Linear-by-Linear Association	,090	1	,765
N of Valid Cases	445		

a. 0 cells (,0%) have expected count less than 5. The minimum expected count is 60,36.

qol * married Crosstabulation

Count

		married		Total
		Unmarried	Married	
qol	low	66	55	121
	medium	53	119	172
	high	37	115	152
Total		156	289	445

Chi-Square Tests

	Value	df	Asymp. Sig. (2-sided)
Pearson Chi-Square	29,211[a]	2	,000
Likelihood Ratio	28,623	2	,000
Linear-by-Linear Association	25,718	1	,000
N of Valid Cases	445		

a. 0 cells (,0%) have expected count less than 5. The minimum expected count is 42,42.

qol * lifestyle Crosstabulation

Count

		lifestyle		
		Inactive	Active	Total
qol	low	43	78	121
	medium	110	62	172
	high	86	66	152
Total		239	206	445

Chi-Square Tests

	Value	df	Asymp. Sig. (2-sided)
Pearson Chi-Square	23,835[a]	2	,000
Likelihood Ratio	24,035	2	,000
Linear-by-Linear Association	10,288	1	,001
N of Valid Cases	445		

a. 0 cells (,0%) have expected count less than 5. The minimum expected count is 56,01.

Except for gender, all of the predictors were statistically significant. Interactions between outcome and factor were, thus, assessed in the traditional efficacy analysis. To better account for nonlinear relationships, neural networks may be more appropriate than traditional testing, and radial basis neural networks was applied.

16.4 Neural Networks for Efficacy Analysis

Radial basis functions may better than multilayer neural network, predict medical data, because it uses a Gaussian activation function, but it is rarely used. This chapter is to assess its performance in clinical research. The SPSS module Neural Networks is used for training and outcome prediction. It uses XML (exTended Markup Language) files to store the neural network. Start by opening the data file in SPSS statistical software on your computer.

Command

click Transform. . . .click Random Number Generators. . . .click Set Starting Point. . . . click Fixed Value (2000000). . . .click OK. . . .click Analyze. . . . Neural Networks . . . .Radial Basis Function. . . .Dependent Variables: enter qol . . . .Factors: age, gender, married, lifestyle. . . .Partitions: Training 7. . . .Test 3. . . .Holdout 0. . . . click Output: mark Description. . . .Diagram. . . . Model summary. . . .Predicted by observed chart. . . .Case processing summary . . . .click Save: mark Save predicted value of category for each dependent variable. . . .automatically generate unique names . . . .click Export. . . .mark Export synaptic weights estimates to XML file. . . .click Browse. . . .File Name: enter "exportradialbasisnn" and save in the appropriate folder of your computer. . . .click OK.

The output warns, that, in the testing sample, some cases have been excluded from analysis, because of values not occurring in the training sample.

The next page graphs are in the output, and they give the radial basis neural network architecture. It has 6 hidden layers and shows, that neurons, after having received a signal beyond some threshold, propagates it forward to the next layer.

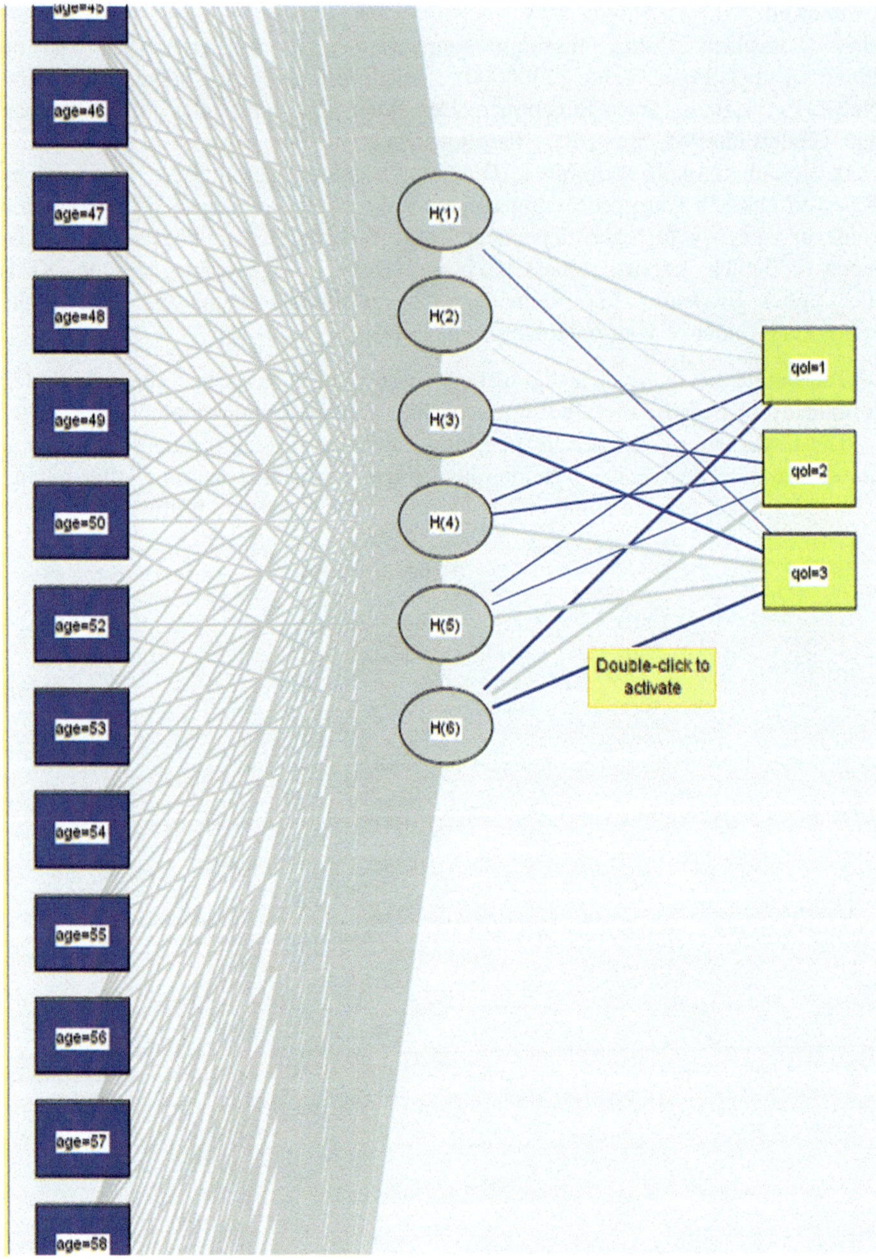
age=46
age=47
age=48
age=49
age=50
age=52
age=53
age=54
age=55
age=56
age=57
age=58
H(1)
H(2)
H(3)
H(4)
H(5)
H(6)
qol=1
qol=2
qol=3
Double-click to activate

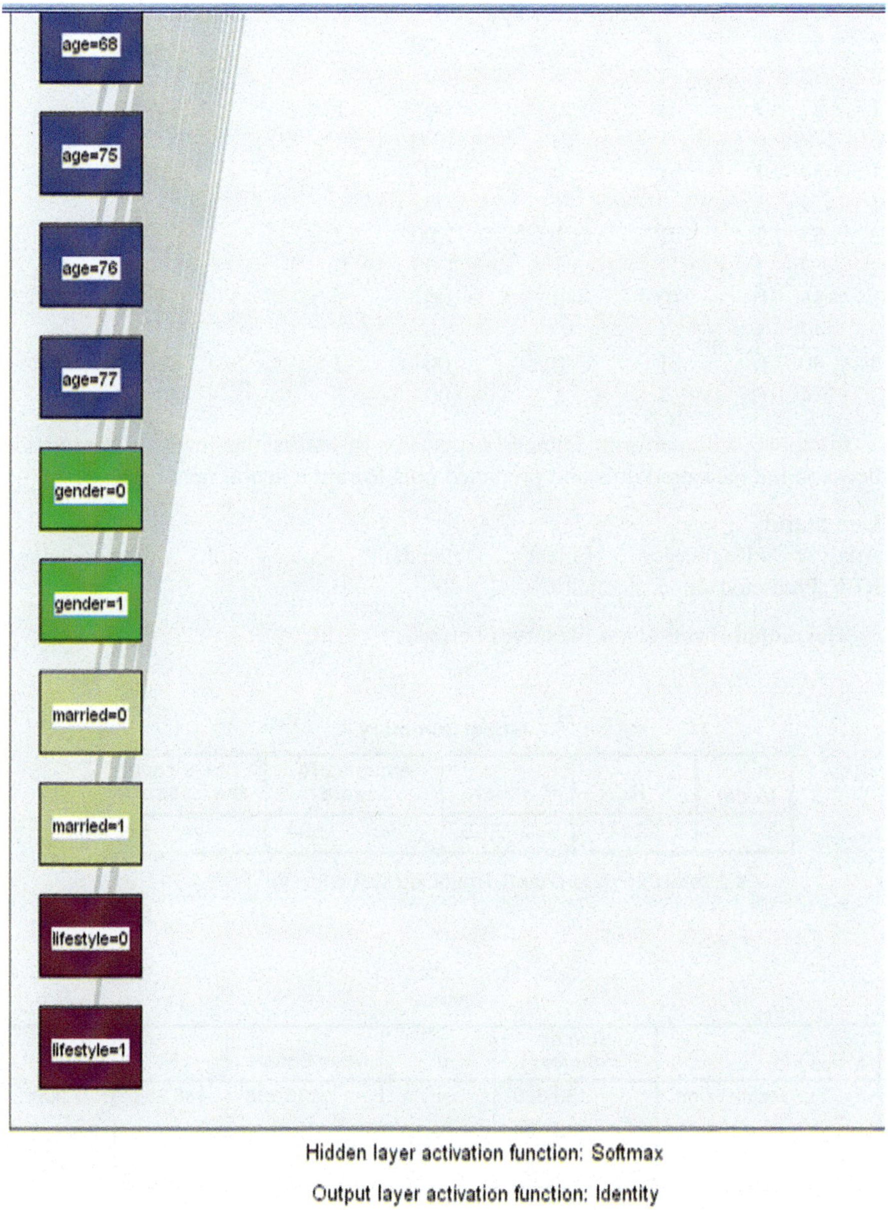

The above graph shows, that, not only age, but also gender, married, and lifestyle are included in the radial basis neural network.

Minimizing the output sheets, the data view screen shows the data file with again a novel variable entitled RBF_PredictedValue. The values, here, are much the same as the measured qols.

qol	age	gender	married	lifestyle	agelevel	RBF_PredictedValue
2	55	1	0	0	1,00	2
2	32	1	1	1	,00	2
1	27	1	1	0	,00	1
3	77	0	1	0	1,00	3
1	34	1	1	0	,00	1
1	35	1	0	1	,00	1
2	57	1	1	1	1,00	2
2	57	1	1	1	1,00	2
1	35	0	0	0	,00	1
2	42	1	1	0	,00	2
3	30	0	1	0	,00	2
1	34	0	1	1	,00	3

First, we will perform a linear regression to assess the level of association between the measured qols and predicted qols from the neural network.

Command

Analyze. . . .Regression. . . .Linear. . . .Dependent: enter qol. . . .Independent(s): RBF_PredictedValue. . . .click OK.

The output sheets show the tables below.

Model Summary

Model	R	R Square	Adjusted R Square	Std. Error of the Estimate
1	,711[a]	,505	,504	,552

a. Predictors: (Constant), Predicted Value for qol

ANOVA[b]

Model		Sum of Squares	df	Mean Square	F	Sig.
1	Regression	136,888	1	136,888	448,686	,000[a]
	Residual	133,933	439	,305		
	Total	270,821	440			

a. Predictors: (Constant), Predicted Value for qol
b. Dependent Variable: qol

Coefficients[a]

Model		Unstandardized Coefficients		Standardized Coefficients	t	Sig.
		B	Std. Error	Beta		
1	(Constant)	,448	,081		5,531	,000
	Predicted Value for qol	,773	,037	,711	21,182	,000

a. Dependent Variable: qol

The linear correlation is very significant, but the Pearson linear coefficient is only 71%. The r square is only 51%, and, so, the predictor only predicts the measured qol by 51%, a pretty poor result.

The linear regression model does not fit the data very well, because the data have a predominantly discrete character. A multinomial regression model may give a better fit. In SPSS the underneath commands are adequate for the purpose.

Command

Analyze....Regression....Multinomial Logistic....Dependent; enter qol....Independent (s): enter RBF_PredictedValue....click OK.

The output sheets show the tables below.

Likelihood Ratio Tests

Effect	Model Fitting Criteria	Likelihood Ratio Tests		
	-2 Log Likelihood of Reduced Model	Chi-Square	df	Sig.
Intercept	25,638[a]	,000	0	.
RBF_PredictedValue	388,337	362,698	4	,000

The chi-square statistic is the difference in -2 log-likelihoods between the final model and a reduced model. The reduced model is formed by omitting an effect from the final model. The null hypothesis is that all parameters of that effect are 0.

a. This reduced model is equivalent to the final model because omitting the effect does not increase the degrees of freedom.

Parameter Estimates

qol[a]		B	Std. Error	Wald	df	Sig.	Exp(B)	95% Confidence Interval for Exp (B)	
								Lower Bound	Upper Bound
low	Intercept	-3,350	,509	43,366	1	,000			
	[RBF_PredictedValue=1]	5,429	,609	79,397	1	,000	228,000	69,068	752,644
	[RBF_PredictedValue=2]	3,629	,567	40,953	1	,000	37,661	12,395	114,430
	[RBF_PredictedValue=3]	0[b]	.	.	0	.	.	.	.
medium	Intercept	-1,740	,242	51,542	1	,000			
	[RBF_PredictedValue=1]	1,047	,599	3,057	1	,080	2,850	,881	9,219
	[RBF_PredictedValue=2]	3,371	,319	111,987	1	,000	29,111	15,592	54,351
	[RBF_PredictedValue=3]	0[b]	.	.	0	.	.	.	.

a. The reference category is: high.
b. This parameter is set to zero because it is redundant.

Obviously, the radial basis neural network predictions of both the low and medium qol levels were statistically significant up to $p < 0.0001$, the best level there is.

Obviously, the multinomial regression model provided a better fit of the neural network predicted to the measured qol, than the linear model did. And the radial basis neural network was, thus, a very good model for making predictions of qol from the combination of predicting variables, age, gender, being married, and lifestyle. In extras.springer.com we have a novel data file entitled "exportradialbasisnn". This program can be used to learn our computer making predictions about future patients, and we will test, whether it works. First, a new data file from 6 future patients is recruited and entered in SPSS statistical software as a New File.

age	gender	married	lifestyle
77	1	1	0
67	1	1	0
65	0	1	0
34	1	0	0
64	0	0	1
40	1	1	0
34	1	0	1

We want to make predictions about the quality of life of these patients. We will make use of the above exported learning file entitled "exportradialbasisnn". For the purpose the Utilities and the Scoring Wizard options must be used.

Command

Utilities....click Scoring Wizard....click Browse....click Select....Folder: enter the exportradialbasisnn.xml file....click Select....in Scoring Wizard click Next.... click Use value substitution....click Next....click Finish.

The underneath data file gives the predicted qols now present in the data view screen

age	gender	married	lifestyle	RBF_PredictedValue
77	1	1	0	1
67	1	1	0	1
65	0	1	0	1
34	1	0	0	1
64	0	0	1	1
40	1	1	0	1
34	1	0	1	1

All of the six new patients are here put in the qol 1 level by the computer.

Conclusion: radial basis neural networks can be readily trained to provide qol values of individual patients.

16.5 Discussion

Lifestyle levels can be considered as interventions in a life, and clinical trials, assessing the different effects of these levels on an outcome like quality of life, can be considered as interventional clinical trials, pretty much similar to controlled drug trials. The effect of discrete predictors on health levels are traditionally analyzed with crosstabs and chi-square tests. In contrast, to better account for nonlinear relationships, neural networks may be more appropriate than traditional testing. Radial basis functions (RBFs), as applied in radial basis neural networks, is equivalent to Gaussian kernel regresssion. It may, better than multilayer perceptron neural network, predict medical data, because it uses a Gaussian activation function, but it is rarely used. This chapter was to assess its performance in clinical research. Quality of life is multidimensional, and factors like age, gender, being married, lifestyle may be independent determinants, although maybe rather in a nonlinear and categorical than linear way. A radial basis neural network can be adequately applied to predict the effect of the above factors on qol.

In this chapter the traditional efficacy analysis consisted of discretized continuous predictors, and 3 × 2 crosstabs with 3 × 2 chi-square statistics, and the machine learning analyses included neural networks. The machine learning analyses provided better sensitivity of testing, and were more informative.

16.6 References

To readers requesting more background, theoretical and mathematical information of computations given, several textbooks complementary to the current production and also written by the same authors are available:

Statistics applied to clinical studies 5th edition, 2012,
Machine learning in medicine a complete overview, 2015,
SPSS for starters and 2nd levelers 2nd edition, 2015,
Clinical data analysis on a pocket calculator 2nd edition, 2016,
Understanding clinical data analysis from published research, 2016,
Modern meta-analysis, 2017,
Regression analysis in clinical research, 2018,
Modern Bayesian statistics in clinical research, 2018.
The analysis of safety data of drug trials an update, 2019.

All of them have been edited by Springer Heidelberg Germany.

Chapter 17
Ensembled-Accuracies for Efficacy Analysis

Contents

Abstract In a 200 septic-patient random sample, the effect of laboratory values on the risk of death was tested, both traditionally, and with the help of machine learning.

Traditional efficacy analysis consisted of

discretization of continuous predictors,
crosstabs and chi-square statistics,
multiple binary logistic regressions.

Machine learning efficacy analysis consisted of ensembled-accuracy methods.

The machine learning methods provided better sensitivity of testing, and were more informative.

Keywords Clinical trials · Traditional efficacy analysis · Machine learning efficacy analysis · Ensembled-accuracy methods

T. J. Cleophas, A. H. Zwinderman, *Efficacy Analysis in Clinical Trials an Update*,
https://doi.org/10.1007/978-3-030-19918-0_17

17.1 Introduction

Patients with sepsis were assessed for factors of death. Surrogates for the factors were various laboratory values of hepatic, renal, and inflammatory functions. The continuous laboratory values were turned into discrete ones with the help of the transform commands of SPSS statistical software. As cut-off for transform, means were applied. The data file is entitled "ensembledmodelbinary", and is in extras.springer.com. A traditional efficacy analysis consisted of multiple 2 × 2 chi-square tests with the laboratory values as predictors and the deaths as outcome. Accuracies of the predictors, measured as true positive and true negative fractions, and average accuracies were not given. For that purpose other methods must be used, like Bayesian networks, cluster analyses, neural networks, or, even better, ensembled procedures including ensembled outcomes of best fit analysis models. The latter methodology will be explained underneath, and tested against the traditional efficacy analysis. Traditional efficacy analysis will consist of discretized continuous predictors, crosstabs and chi-square statistics, and multiple binary logistic regressions.

17.2 Data Example

A 200 patients' data file includes 11 variables consistent of patients' laboratory values and their subsequent outcome (death or alive). Only the first 12 patients are shown underneath. The entire data file is in extras.springer.com, and is entitled "ensembledmodelbinary".

Death	ggt	asat	alat	bili	ureum	creat	c-clear	esr	crp	leucos
,00	20,00	23,00 34,00	2,00	3,40	89,00	−111,00	2,00	2,00	5,00	
,00	14,00	21,00	33,00	3,00	2,00	67,00	−112,00	7,00	3,00	6,00
,00	30,00	35,00	32,00	4,00	5,60	58,00	−116,00	8,00	4,00	4,00
,00	35,00	34,00	40,00	4,00	6,00	76,00	−110,00	6,00	5,00	7,00
,00	23,00	33,00	22,00	4,00	6,10	95,00	−120,00	9,00	6,00	6,00
,00	26,00	31,00	24,00	3,00	5,40	78,00	−132,00	8,00	4,00	8,00
,00	15,00	29,00	26,00	2,00	5,30	47,00	−120,00	12,00	5,00	5,00
,00	13,00	26,00	24,00	1,00	6,30	65,00	−132,00	13,00	6,00	6,00
,00	26,00	27,00	27,00	4,00	6,00	97,00	−112,00	14,00	6,00	7,00
,00	34,00	25,00	13,00	3,00	4,00	67,00	−125,00	15,00	7,00	6,00
,00	32,00	26,00	24,00	3,00	3,60	58,00	−110,00	13,00	8,00	6,00
,00	21,00	13,00	15,00	3,00	3,60	69,00	−102,00	12,00	2,00	4,00

Variable
0.0001 death = death yes no (0 = no)
0.0002 ggt = gamma glutamyl transferase (u/l)
0.0003 asat = aspartate aminotransferase (u/l)
0.0004 alat = alanine aminotransferase (u/l)
0.0005 bili = bilirubine (micromol/l)
0.0006 ureum = ureum (mmol/l)
0.0007 creat= creatinine (mmicromol/l)
0.0008 c-clear = creatinine clearance (ml/min)
0.0009 esr = erythrocyte sedimentation rate (mm)
0.0010 crp = c-reactive protein (mg/l)
0.0011 leucos = leucocyte count (.10^9 /l)

17.3 Traditional Efficacy Analysis

Traditional efficacy analysis consists of t-tests for continuous outcomes and chi-square tests for discrete outcomes. In Sect. 1.12, Chap. 1, the use of regression analyses for efficacy analyses is discussed, and in Sect. 1.13 the use of clinical trials for the assessment of causal health effects of factors other than medicines is discussed. For example, effects of interventions like angioplasties, surgeries, renal transplants etc. Many more factors can be tested in clinical trials, for example,

age factors
psychological factors
social factors
physical factors
economical factors,
and, any factor with a supposedly causal effect on health or sickness.

In the current chapter start by opening the data file in your computer with SPSS statistical software installed.

Command

click Analyze. . . .Descriptive Statistics. . . .Descriptives. . . .Variable(s). . . .enter Var 00001 to 00011. . . .click OK.

The means and standard deviations are given in the output.

Descriptive Statistics

	N	Minimum	Maximum	Mean	Std. Deviation
gammagt	200	2,00	2300,00	200,4950	349,59912
asat	200	3,00	1980,00	194,3950	335,60735
alat	200	2,00	1500,00	190,5400	308,25185
bili	200	1,00	400,00	62,0900	94,28793
ureum	200	2,00	98,00	15,2525	19,02840
creatinine	200	47,00	865,00	192,8100	190,15517
creatinine clearance	200	-132,00	-4,00	-80,1200	41,94188
esr	200	2,00	180,00	38,9200	39,69170
c-reactive protein	200	2,00	243,00	23,2400	35,37839
leucos	200	2,00	30,00	12,0450	7,75912
Valid N (listwise)	200				

We will apply the means from the above table for cut-offs for the purpose of discretization of the continuous variables.

Command

Transform. . . .Compute Variable. . . .Target Variable: write the term ggt. . . .Numeric Expression: enter gammagt. . . .click ">" from the blue field. . . .then click "200". . . . click OK.

In the data view screen now a novel variable entitled ggt is observed. We will test the significance of difference between the effect of two groups of predictors on numbers of deaths.

		death no	death yes
group 1	ggt > 200	a	b
group 2	ggt < 200	c	d

a to d = number of patients per cell.

For that purpose a chi-square test of the above 2 × 2 crosstab will be performed. Command.

Command

Analyze. . . .Descriptives. . . .Crosstabs. . . .Rows: enter ggt. . . .Column (s). . . .click Statistics. . . .mark chi-square. . . .click Continue. . . .click OK.

The tables below are in the output sheets.

ggt * death Crosstabulation

Count

		death		Total
		,00	1,00	
ggt	,00	107	41	148
	1,00	0	52	52
Total		107	93	200

Chi-Square Tests

	Value	df	Asymp. Sig. (2-sided)	Exact Sig. (2-sided)	Exact Sig. (1-sided)
Pearson Chi-Square	80,849[a]	1	,000		
Continuity Correction[b]	77,969	1	,000		
Likelihood Ratio	101,602	1	,000		
Fisher's Exact Test				,000	,000
Linear-by-Linear Association	80,444	1	,000		
N of Valid Cases	200				

a. 0 cells (,0%) have expected count less than 5. The minimum expected count is 24,18.
b. Computed only for a 2x2 table

No deaths were in the cell with ggt < 200. Although the chi-square is flawed with cells smaller than 5 subjects, the p-values of 0.000 suggests that ggt is a very strong surrogate factor of death. In the same way all of the surrogate factors were applied for testing.

All of the p-values were < 0.000. The chi-square values were very high.

laboratory values	chi-square values	p-values
gamma gt	80.8	0.000
asat	88.0	0.000
alat	83.0	0.000
bili	99.6	0.000
ureum	85.8	0.000
creatinine	77.9	0.000
creatinine clearance	137.7	0.000
esr	102	0.000
c-reactive protein	90.3	
leucos	148.4	

The best chi-squares were produced by the leucocyte counts and the creatinine clearances. The analyses were univariate, and, so, confoundings and interactions of the predictors on the outcome were not taken into account.

A multiple logistic regression with all of the undiscretized predictors was performed.

Command

Analyze. . . .Regression. . . .Binary Logistic. . . .Dependent: enter death. . . .Covariate (s): enter: all of the original predictors. . . .click OK.

In the output only 3 predictors remained independent: Var 00005 (bili), 00010 (creactp), 00011 (leuco).

Variables in the Equation

		B	S.E.	Wald	df	Sig.	Exp(B)
Step 1[a]	VAR00002	,020	,019	1,141	1	,285	1,020
	VAR00003	,003	,017	,034	1	,854	1,003
	VAR00004	,001	,015	,002	1	,965	1,001
	VAR00005	,038	,017	5,237	1	,022	1,039
	VAR00006	-,172	,112	2,350	1	,125	,842
	VAR00007	,001	,008	,016	1	,901	1,001
	VAR00008	-,036	,034	1,147	1	,284	,964
	VAR00009	-,021	,049	,187	1	,665	,979
	VAR00010	-,068	,033	4,270	1	,039	,934
	VAR00011	1,236	,395	9,781	1	,002	3,442
	Constant	-17,739	6,609	7,205	1	,007	,000

a. Variable(s) entered on step 1: VAR00002, VAR00003, VAR00004, VAR00005, VAR00006, VAR00007, VAR00008, VAR00009, VAR00010, VAR00011.

A multiple logistic regression with all of the discretized predictors was, subsequently, performed.

Command

Analyze. . . .Regression. . . .Binary Logistic. . . .Dependent: enter death. . . .Covariate (s): enter: all of the discretized predictors. . . .click OK.

In the output only 2 predictors remained independent: creatinine clearance and leucocyte count. But they were significant at better levels of significance than the predictors of the undiscretized analysis was.

Variables in the Equation

		B	S.E.	Wald	df	Sig.	Exp(B)
Step 1[a]	ggt	90,453	6008,584	,000	1	,988	1,919E39
	asat	-10,832	1361,181	,000	1	,994	,000
	alat	57,649	4587,495	,000	1	,990	1,088E25
	bili	1,198	2,654	,204	1	,652	3,313
	ureum	33,467	2837,424	,000	1	,991	3,425E14
	creatinine	-57,013	4142,290	,000	1	,989	,000
	creatinineclearance	-3,729	,823	20,547	1	,000	,024
	esr	33,300	2697,568	,000	1	,990	2,897E14
	creactp	-12,008	1350,962	,000	1	,993	,000
	leuco	3,344	1,093	9,350	1	,002	28,319
	Constant	,121	,610	,040	1	,842	1,129

a. Variable(s) entered on step 1: ggt, asat, alat, bili, ureum, creatinine, creatinineclearance, esr, creactp, leuco.

The traditional efficacy analysis underscored the importance of laboratory values as surrogates for mortality in patients with sepsis. Accuracies of the predictors, measured as true positive and true negative fractions, and average accuracies were, however, not given. For that purpose other methods must be used, like Bayesian networks, cluster analyses, neural networks, or, even better, ensembled procedures including ensembled outcomes of best fit analysis models. The latter methodology will be applied underneath.

17.4 Ensembled Accuracies for Efficacy Analysis

SPSS modeler is a work bench for automatic data mining and modeling. So far it is virtually unused in medicine, and mainly applied by econo-/sociometrists. Automatic modeling of binary outcomes computes the ensembled result of a number of best fit models for a particular data set, and provides better sensitivity than the separate models do.

17.4.1 Step 1 Open SPSS Modeler (14.2)

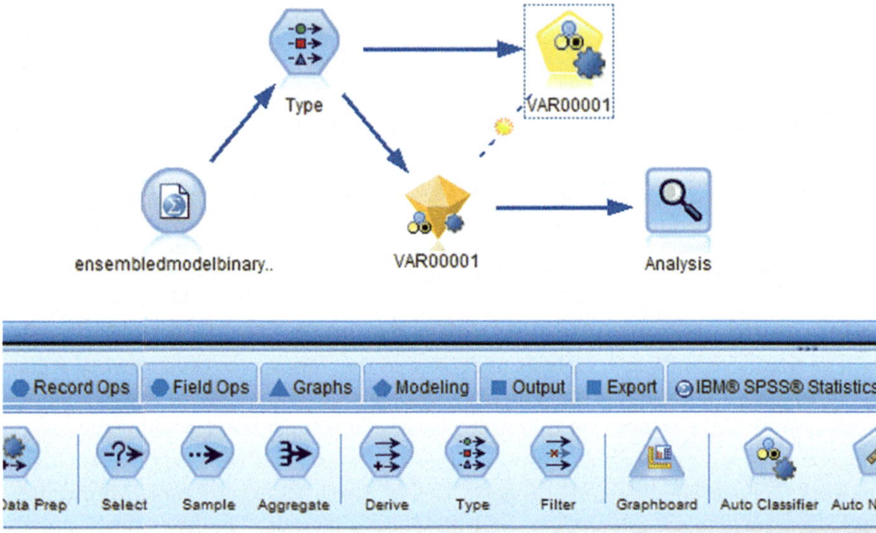

17.4.2 Step 2 the Statistics File Node

The canvas is, initially, blank, and above is given a screen view of the completed ensembled model, otherwise called stream of nodes, which we are going to build. First, in the palettes at the bottom of the screen full of nodes, look and find the **Statistics File node**, and drag it to the canvas, pressing the mouse left side. Double-click on this node. . . .Import file: browse and enter the file "ensembledmodelbinary" . . . .click OK. The graph below shows, that the data file is open for analysis.

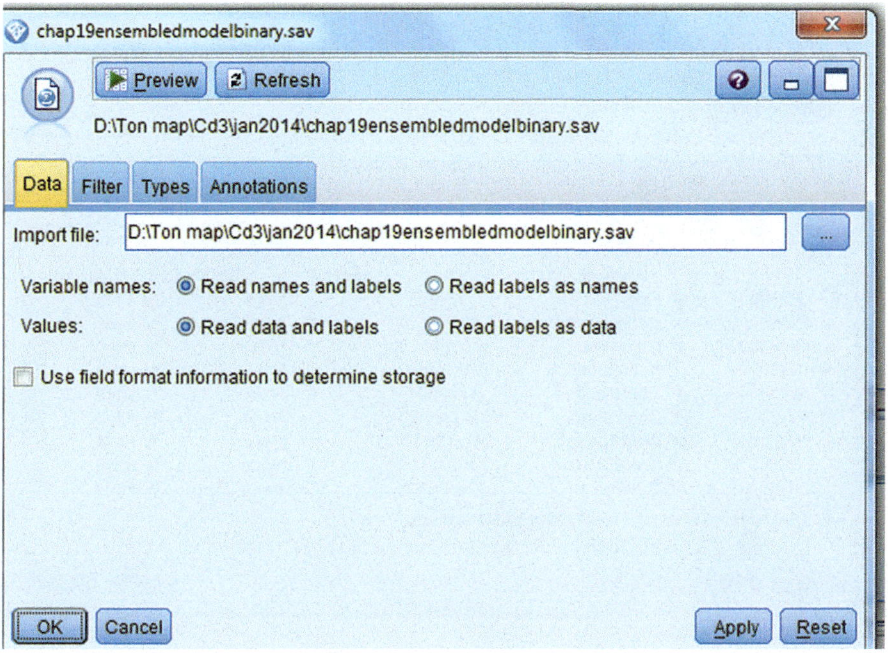

17.4.3 Step 3 the Type Node

In the palette at the bottom of screen find Type node and drag to the canvas. . . .right-click on the Statistics File node. . . .a Connect symbol comes up. . . .click on the Type node. . . .an arrow is displayed. . . .double-click on the Type Node. . . .after a second or two the underneath graph with information from the Type node is observed. Type nodes are used to access the properties of the variables (often called fields here) like type, role, unit etc. in the data file. As shown below, 10 predictor variables (all of them continuous) are appropriately set. However, VAR 00001 (death) is the outcome (= target) variable, and is binary. Click in the row of variable VAR00001 on the measurement column and replace "Continuous" with "Flag". Click Apply and OK. The underneath figure is removed and the canvas is displayed again.

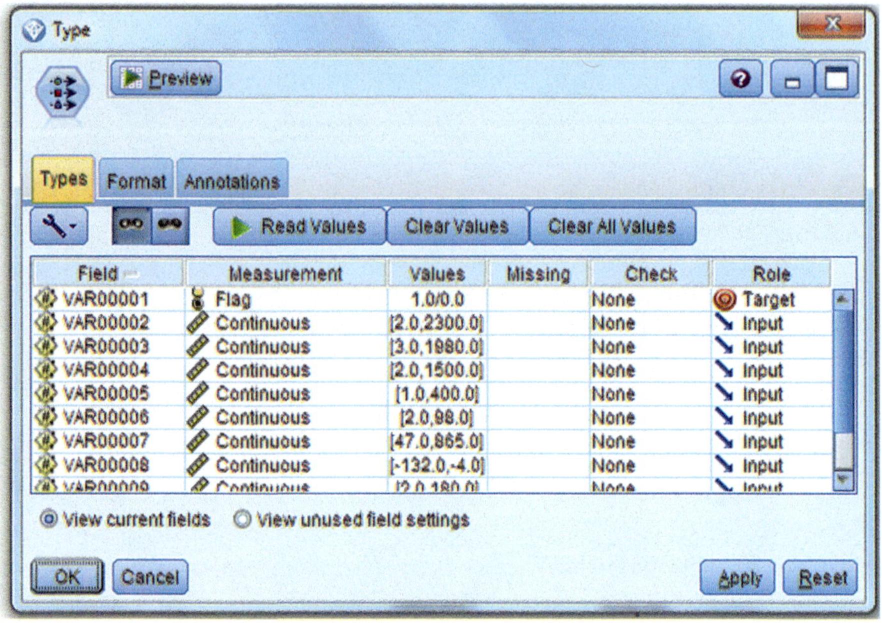

17.4.4 Step 4 the Auto Classifier Node

Now, click the Auto Classifier node and drag to the canvas, and connect with the Type node using the above connect-procedure. Click the Auto Classifier node, and the underneath graph comes up. . . .now click Model. . . .select Lift as Rank model of the various analysis models used. . . . the additional manoeuvres are as indicated below. . . .in Numbers of models to use: type the number 4.

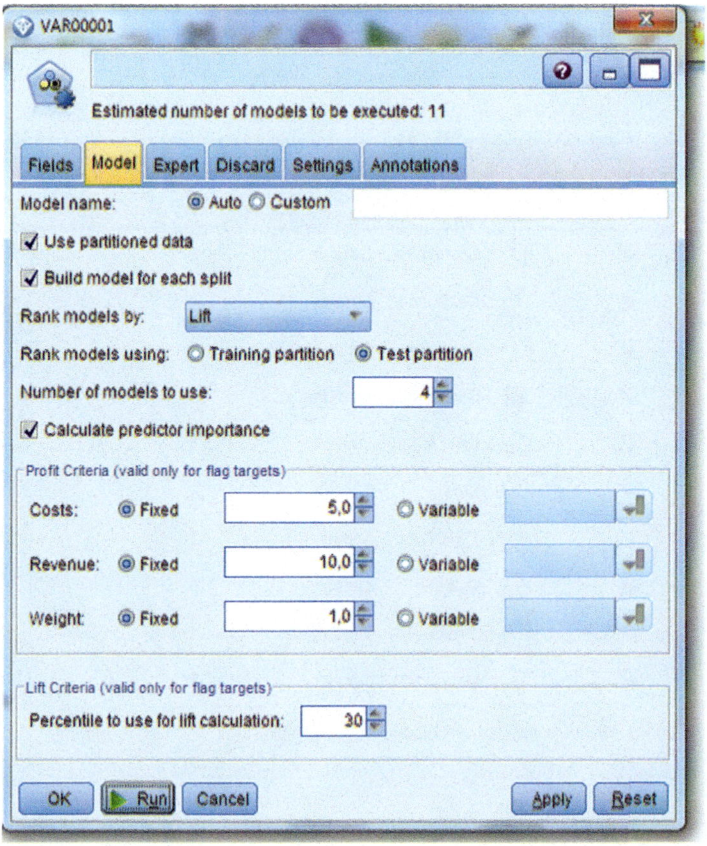

17.4.5 Step 5 the Expert Tab

Then click the Expert tab. It is shown below. Out of 11 statistical models the four best fit ones are selected by SPSS modeler for constructing an ensembled model.

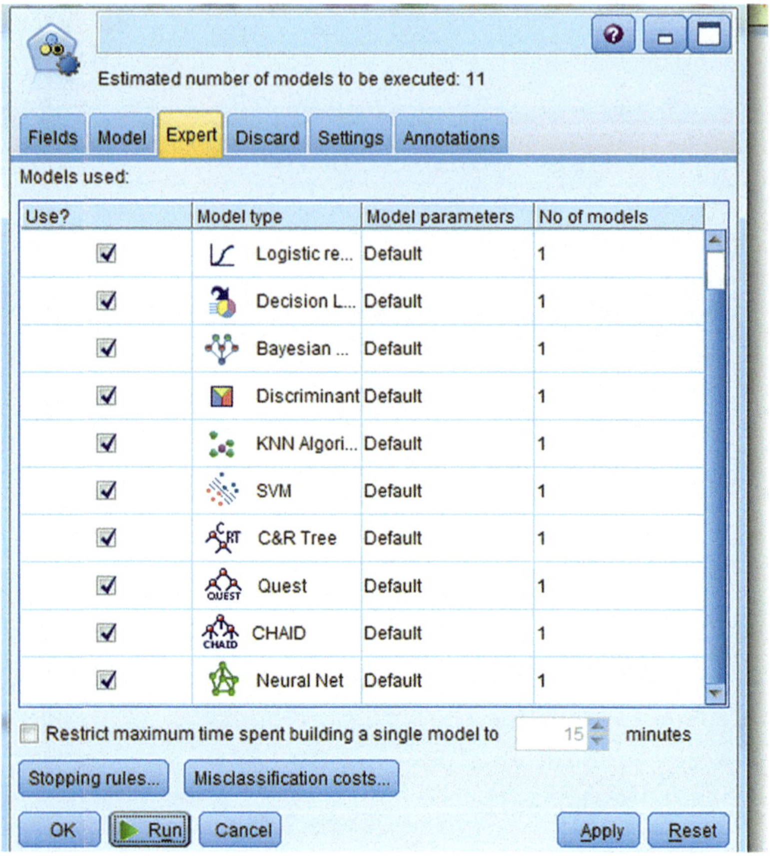

The 11 statistical analysis methods for a flag target (= binary outcome) include:

1/. C5.0 decision tree (C5.0)
2/. Logistic regression (Logist r. . .)
3/. Decision list (Decision. . . .)
4/. Bayesian network (Bayesian. . . .)
5/. Discriminant analysis (Discriminant)
6/. K nearest neighbors algorithm (KNN Alg. . .)
7/. Support vector machine (SVM)
8/. Classification and regression tree (C&R Tree)
9/. Quest decision tree (Quest Tr. . . .)
10/. Chi square automatic interaction detection (CHAID Tree)
11/. Neural network (Neural Net)

17.4.6 Step 6 the Settings Tab

In the above graph click the Settings tab. . . .click the Run button. . . .now a gold nugget is placed on the canvas. . . .click the gold nugget. . . .the model created is shown below.

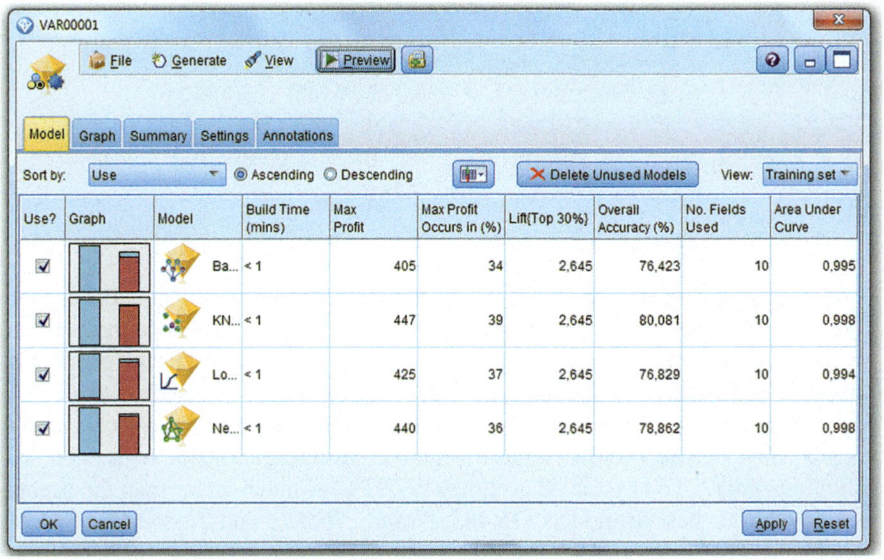

The overall accuracies (%) of the four best fit models are over 0.8, and are, thus, pretty good. We will now perform the ensembled procedure.

17.4.7 Step 7 the Analysis Node

Find in the palettes at the bottom of the screen the Analysis node and drag it to the canvas. With above connect procedure connect it with the gold nugget. . . .click the Analysis node.

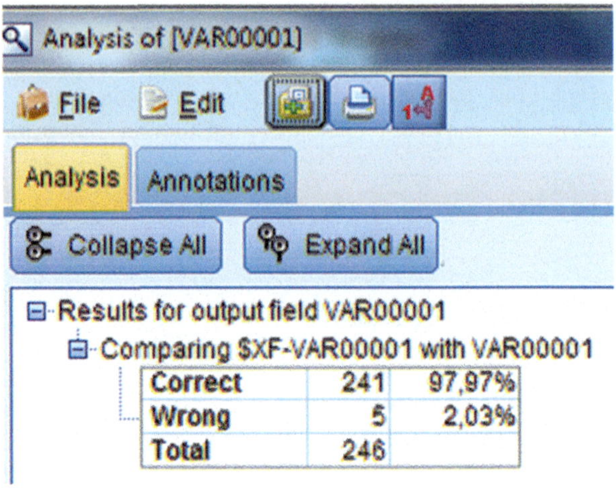

Correct	241	97,97%
Wrong	5	2,03%
Total	246	

The above table is shown and gives the statistics of the ensembled model created. The ensembled outcome is the average accuracy of the accuracies from the four best fit statistical models. In order to prevent overstated certainty due to overfitting, bootstrap aggregating ("bagging") is used. The ensembled outcome (named the $XR-outcome) is compared with the outcomes of the four best fit statistical models, namely, Bayesian network, k Nearest Neighbor clustering, Logistic regression, and Neural network. The ensembled accuracy (97.97%) is much larger than the accuracies of the four best fit models (76,423, 80,081, 76,829, and 78,862 %), and, so, ensembled procedures make sense, because they provide increased precision in the analysis. The computed ensembled model can now be stored in your computer in the form of an SPSS Modeler Stream file for future use. For the readers' convenience it is in extras.springer.com , and entitled "ensembledmodelbinary".

17.5 Discussion

Traditional efficacy analysis with multiple 2 × 2 chi-square tests were tested against ensembled accuracy analysis. As data example, patients with sepsis were assessed for factors of death. Surrogates for the factors were various laboratory values of hepatic, renal, and inflammatory functions. The continuous laboratory values were turned into discrete ones. As cut-off for transform, means were applied. A traditional efficacy analysis consisted of multiple 2 × 2 chi-square tests with the laboratory values as predictors and the deaths as outcome. The traditional efficacy analysis produced very significant effects of predictors on outcome, but accuracies of the predictors, measured as true positive and true negative fractions, and average accuracies were not given. For that purpose machine learning methods had to be used, including Bayesian networks, cluster analyses, neural networks, or, even better, ensembled procedures including the best fit analysis models available. The latter methodology was explained, and tested against the traditional efficacy analysis.

In the example given in this chapter, the ensembled accuracy is larger (97,97%) than the accuracies from the four best fit models (76,423, 80,081, 76,829, and 78,862 %), and so ensembled procedures make sense, because they can provide increased precision in the analysis.

In this chapter the traditional efficacy analysis consisted of discretized continuous predictors, crosstabs and chi-square statistics, and multiple binary logistic regressions, and the machine learning analyses included ensembled accuracy models. The machine learning analyses provided better sensitivity of testing, and were more informative.

17.6 References

To readers requesting more background, theoretical and mathematical information of computations given, several textbooks complementary to the current production and written by the same authors are available:

Statistics applied to clinical studies 5th edition, 2012,
Machine learning in medicine a complete overview, 2015,
SPSS for starters and 2nd levelers 2nd edition, 2015,
Clinical data analysis on a pocket calculator 2nd edition, 2016,
Understanding clinical data analysis from published research, 2016,
Modern meta-analysis, 2017,
Regression analysis in clinical research, 2018,
Modern Bayesian statistics in clinical research, 2018.
The Analysis of Safety Data of Drug Trials, an Update, 2019.

All of them have been edited by Springer Heidelberg Germany.

Chapter 18
Ensembled-Correlations for Efficacy Analysis

Contents

Abstract In a 250 patient self-controlled study, the effects of highly expressed gene polymorphisms on drug efficacy was tested, both traditionally, and with the help of machine learning.

Traditional efficacy analysis consisted of

simple linear regressions,

multiple linear regressions,

Bonferroni's adjustments.

Machine learning efficacy analysis consisted of ensembled-correlation methods.

The machine learning methods provided better sensitivity of testing, and were more informative.

Keywords Clinical trials · Traditional efficacy analysis · Machine learning efficacy analysis · Ensembled-correlation methods

T. J. Cleophas, A. H. Zwinderman, *Efficacy Analysis in Clinical Trials an Update*,
https://doi.org/10.1007/978-3-030-19918-0_18

18.1 Introduction

Automatic modeling of continuous outcomes computes the ensembled result of a number of best fit models for a particular data set, and provides better sensitivity of testing than the separate analysis models do. This chapter is to assess, whether it can be used for efficacy analysis of clinical trials, and to test its performance against that of traditional efficacy analysis, for the purpose. Traditional efficacy analysis will consist of simple linear regressions, multiple linear regressions, and Bonferroni's adjustments.

18.2 Data Example

This chapter will use a 250 patient self-controlled study of drug efficacy scores, measured as differences from baseline. The traditional efficacy analysis used simple linear regressions of highly expressed gene levels versus the drug efficacy scores, and step down multiple linear regressions to identify the best fit combination of highly expressed gene levels. The gene expression levels were scored on a scale of 0–10.

G1	G2	G3	G4	G16	G17	G18	G19	G24	G25	G26	G27	O1	O2	O3	O4
8	8	9	5	7	10	5	6	9	9	6	6	6	7	6	7
9	9	10	9	8	8	7	8	8	9	8	8	8	7	8	7
9	8	8	8	8	9	7	8	9	8	9	9	9	8	8	8
8	9	8	9	6	7	6	4	6	6	5	5	7	7	7	6
10	10	8	10	9	10	10	8	8	9	9	9	8	8	8	7
7	8	8	8	8	7	6	5	7	8	8	7	7	6	6	7
5	5	5	5	5	6	4	5	5	6	6	5	6	5	6	4
9	9	9	9	8	8	8	8	9	8	3	8	8	8	8	8
9	8	9	8	9	8	7	7	7	7	5	8	8	7	6	6
10	10	10	10	10	10	10	10	10	8	8	10	10	10	9	10
2	2	8	5	7	8	8	8	9	3	9	8	7	7	7	6
7	8	8	7	8	6	6	7	8	8	8	7	8	7	8	8
8	9	9	8	10	8	8	7	8	8	9	9	7	7	8	8

Variables G1-27 highly expressed genes estimated from their arrays' normalized ratios

Variables O1-4 drug efficacy scores (mean of sum of the scores is used as composite outcome)

Only the data from the first 13 patients are shown. The entire data file entitled "ensembledmodelscontinuous" can be downloaded from extra.springer.com.

18.3 Traditional Efficacy Analysis

Traditional efficacy analysis consists of t-tests for continuous outcomes and chi-square tests for discrete outcomes. In Sect. 1.12, Chap. 1, the use of regression analyses for efficacy analyses is discussed, and in Sect. 1.13 the use of clinical trials for the assessment of causal health effects of factors other than medicines is discussed. For example, effects of interventions like angioplasties, surgeries, renal transplants etc. Many more factors can be tested in clinical trials, for example,

age factors
psychological factors
social factors
physical factors
economical factors,
and, any factor with a supposedly causal effect on health or sickness.

In the current chapter SPSS statistical software is used for data analysis. Univariate linear regressions will be performed with all of the genes as predictors and the composite drug efficacy score as outcome. Open the data file in your computer mounted with SPSS, and command.

Command

Analyze....Regression....Linear....Dependent: outcome.... Independent: enter the 12 highly expressed genes one by one ....click OK.

In the output sheets the underneath tables are given.

Coefficients[a]

Model		Unstandardized Coefficients		Standardized Coefficients	t	Sig.
		B	Std. Error	Beta		
1	(Constant)	3,627	,547		6,634	,000
	geneone	,421	,068	,364	6,150	,000

a. Dependent Variable: outcome

Coefficients[a]

Model		Unstandardized Coefficients		Standardized Coefficients	t	Sig.
		B	Std. Error	Beta		
1	(Constant)	2,457	,454		5,408	,000
	genetwo	,571	,057	,539	10,077	,000

a. Dependent Variable: outcome

Coefficients[a]

Model		Unstandardized Coefficients		Standardized Coefficients	t	Sig.
		B	Std. Error	Beta		
1	(Constant)	1,833	,461		3,975	,000
	genethree	,642	,057	,583	11,293	,000

a. Dependent Variable: outcome

Coefficients[a]

Model		Unstandardized Coefficients		Standardized Coefficients	t	Sig.
		B	Std. Error	Beta		
1	(Constant)	3,510	,621		5,651	,000
	genefour	,432	,077	,334	5,577	,000

a. Dependent Variable: outcome

Coefficients[a]

Model		Unstandardized Coefficients		Standardized Coefficients	t	Sig.
		B	Std. Error	Beta		
1	(Constant)	2,313	,300		7,714	,000
	genesixteen	,652	,041	,714	16,038	,000

a. Dependent Variable: outcome

Coefficients[a]

Model		Unstandardized Coefficients		Standardized Coefficients	t	Sig.
		B	Std. Error	Beta		
1	(Constant)	1,457	,414		3,516	,001
	geneseventeen	,709	,052	,652	13,525	,000

a. Dependent Variable: outcome

Coefficients[a]

Model		Unstandardized Coefficients		Standardized Coefficients	t	Sig.
		B	Std. Error	Beta		
1	(Constant)	3,343	,367		9,113	,000
	geneeighteen	,502	,049	,542	10,153	,000

a. Dependent Variable: outcome

Coefficients[a]

Model		Unstandardized Coefficients		Standardized Coefficients	t	Sig.
		B	Std. Error	Beta		
1	(Constant)	3,066	,284		10,807	,000
	genenineteen	,595	,041	,673	14,337	,000

a. Dependent Variable: outcome

Coefficients[a]

Model		Unstandardized Coefficients		Standardized Coefficients	t	Sig.
		B	Std. Error	Beta		
1	(Constant)	3,696	,293		12,608	,000
	genetwentyfour	,450	,039	,596	11,675	,000

a. Dependent Variable: outcome

Coefficients[a]

Model		Unstandardized Coefficients		Standardized Coefficients	t	Sig.
		B	Std. Error	Beta		
1	(Constant)	4,679	,445		10,504	,000
	genetwentyfive	,302	,058	,314	5,199	,000

a. Dependent Variable: outcome

Coefficients[a]

Model		Unstandardized Coefficients		Standardized Coefficients	t	Sig.
		B	Std. Error	Beta		
1	(Constant)	3,937	,276		14,251	,000
	genetwentysix	,438	,038	,592	11,566	,000

a. Dependent Variable: outcome

Coefficients[a]

Model		Unstandardized Coefficients		Standardized Coefficients	t	Sig.
		B	Std. Error	Beta		
1	(Constant)	5,117	,420		12,193	,000
	genetwentyseven	,236	,053	,273	4,464	,000

a. Dependent Variable: outcome

Obviously, all of the above univariate linear regressions were statistically very significant with t-values from 3.5 to 16.0. However, dependencies between the predicting gene expression levels were not accounted in the analyses so far. Therefore, a step down multiple linear regression was in the protocol, and was, subsequently performed.

Command

Analyze....Regression....Linear....Dependent: outcome.... Independent: enter the 12 highly expressed genes simultaneously ....click OK.

In the output sheets the underneath table was given.

Coefficients[a]

Model		Unstandardized Coefficients		Standardized Coefficients	t	Sig.
		B	Std. Error	Beta		
1	(Constant)	,538	,467		1,154	,250
	geneone	-,014	,060	-,012	-,228	,820
	genetwo	,047	,071	,045	,664	,507
	genethree	,032	,072	,029	,438	,662
	genefour	,069	,062	,053	1,107	,269
	genesixteen	,225	,054	,246	4,148	,000
	geneseventeen	,248	,063	,228	3,962	,000
	geneeighteen	,081	,048	,087	1,687	,093
	genenineteen	,205	,049	,232	4,225	,000
	genetwentyfour	,102	,046	,135	2,219	,027
	genetwentyfive	-,052	,045	-,054	-1,159	,248
	genetwentysix	,089	,045	,120	1,979	,049
	genetwentyseven	-,136	,042	-,157	-3,225	,001

a. Dependent Variable: outcome

The number of statistically significant p-values, indicated here with Sig. ($p < 0.10$) was 7 out of 12. In order to improve this result, the insignificant predictors were subsequently deleted from the model. And the same commands were given once more. This left us with the model in the underneath table.

Coefficients[a]

Model		Unstandardized Coefficients		Standardized Coefficients	t	Sig.
		B	Std. Error	Beta		
1	(Constant)	,885	,350		2,528	,012
	genesixteen	,238	,052	,261	4,563	,000
	geneseventeen	,254	,062	,234	4,115	,000
	geneeighteen	,101	,047	,109	2,158	,032
	genenineteen	,222	,047	,251	4,716	,000
	genetwentyfour	,101	,046	,134	2,229	,027
	genetwentysix	,081	,043	,110	1,865	,063
	genetwentyseven	-,136	,040	-,158	-3,408	,001

a. Dependent Variable: outcome

In the model 5 insignificant predictors were deleted, and 7 significant ones were maintained. Many very independent determinants were, thus, maintained in the final model, although multiple testing was not yet taken into account.

With Bonferroni correction for multiple testing the rejection type I error (alpha) of 0.05 should be reduced to with number of statistical tests of $k = 7$

$$\begin{aligned} \text{alpha corrected} &= \text{alpha } x[2/k(k-1)] \\ &= 0.05x\ (2/(7\ x\ 6) \\ &= 0.0024 \end{aligned}$$

This would mean, that the gene eighteen, twenty-four and twenty-six were not statistically significant anymore.

18.4 Ensembled-Correlations for Efficacy Analysis

We will use SPSS modeler. It is a work bench for automatic data mining and modeling. So far it is virtually unused in medicine, and mainly applied by econo-/ sociometrics. Automatic modeling of continuous outcomes computes the ensembled result of a number of best fit models for a particular data set, and may provide even better sensitivity than the separate models do.

The expression of a cluster of genes can be used as a functional unit to predict the efficacy of cytostatic treatment. Can ensembled modeling with three best fit statistical models provide better precision of testing, than the separate analysis with single statistical models does.

The above 250 patients' data file is used once more. It includes 28 variables consistent of patients' gene expression levels and their drug efficacy scores. The data file is slightly different from the above data file, because, instead of 4 separate outcome variables, a single composite outcome called outcome score is now given. It is in extras.springer.com, and is entitled "optscaling". All of the variables were standardized by scoring them on 11 points linear scales. The following genes were highly expressed: the genes 1–4, 16–19, and 24–27.

G1	G2	G3	G4	G16	G17	G18	G19	G24	G25	G26	G27	O
8,00	8,00	9,00	5,00	7,00	10,00	5,00	6,00	9,00	9,00	6,00	6,00	7,00
9,00	9,00	10,00	9,00	8,00	8,00	7,00	8,00	8,00	9,00	8,00	8,00	7,00
9,00	8,00	8,00	8,00	8,00	9,00	7,00	8,00	9,00	8,00	9,00	9,00	8,00
8,00	9,00	8,00	9,00	6,00	7,00	6,00	4,00	6,00	6,00	5,00	5,00	7,00
10,00	10,00	8,00	10,00	9,00	10,00	10,00	8,00	8,00	9,00	9,00	9,00	8,00
7,00	8,00	8,00	8,00	8,00	7,00	6,00	5,00	7,00	8,00	8,00	7,00	6,00
5,00	5,00	5,00	5,00	5,00	6,00	4,00	5,00	5,00	6,00	6,00	5,00	5,00
9,00	9,00	9,00	9,00	8,00	8,00	8,00	8,00	9,00	8,00	3,00	8,00	8,00
9,00	8,00	9,00	8,00	9,00	8,00	7,00	7,00	7,00	7,00	5,00	8,00	7,00
10,00	10,00	10,00	10,00	10,00	10,00	10,00	10,00	10,00	8,00	8,00	10,00	10,00
2,00	2,00	8,00	5,00	7,00	8,00	8,00	8,00	9,00	3,00	9,00	8,00	7,00
7,00	8,00	8,00	7,00	8,00	6,00	6,00	7,00	8,00	8,00	8,00	7,00	7,00

G = gene (gene expression levels), O = outcome (score)

18.4.1 Step 1 Open SPSS Modeler (14.2)

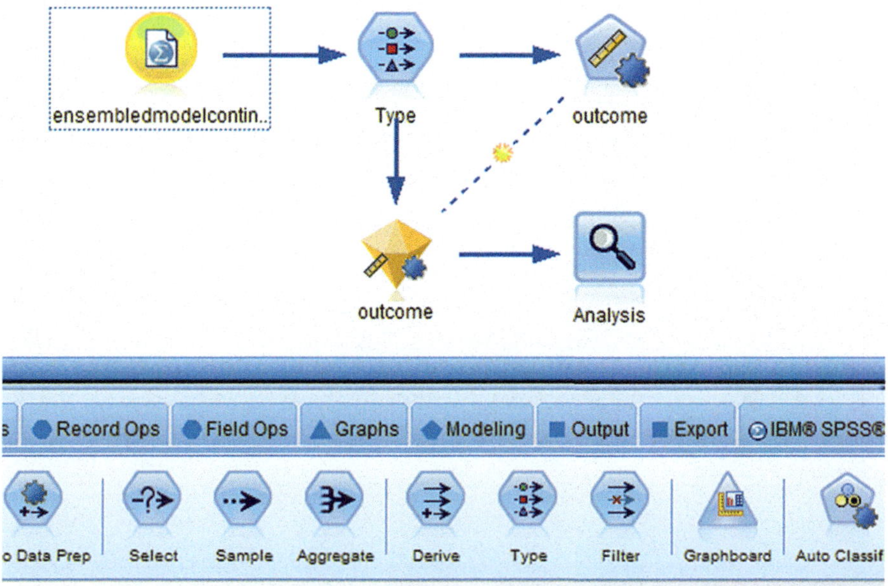

18.4.2 Step 2 the Statistics File Node

The canvas is, initially, blank, and above a screen view is of the final "completed ensemble" model, otherwise called stream of nodes, which we are going to build. First, in the palettes at the bottom of the screen full of nodes, look and find the **Statistics File node**, and drag it to the canvas. Double-click on it. . . .Import file: browse and enter the file "ensembledmodelcontinuous" . . . .click OK. The graph below shows that the data file is open for analysis.

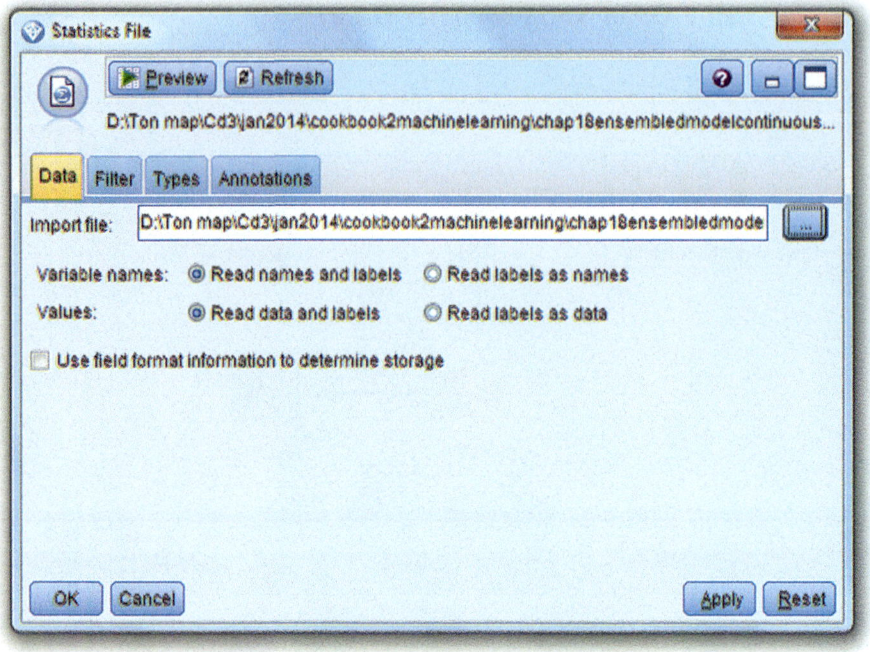

18.4.3 Step 3 the Type Node

In the palette at the bottom of screen find Type node and drag to the canvas. . . .right-click on the Statistics File node. . . .a Connect symbol comes up. . . .click on the Type node. . . .an arrow is displayed. . . .double-click on the Type Node. . . .after a second or two the underneath graph with information from the Type node is observed. Type nodes are used to access the properties of the variables (often called fields here) like type, role, unit etc. in the data file. As shown below, the variables are appropriately set: 14 predictor variables, 1 outcome (= target) variable, all of them continuous.

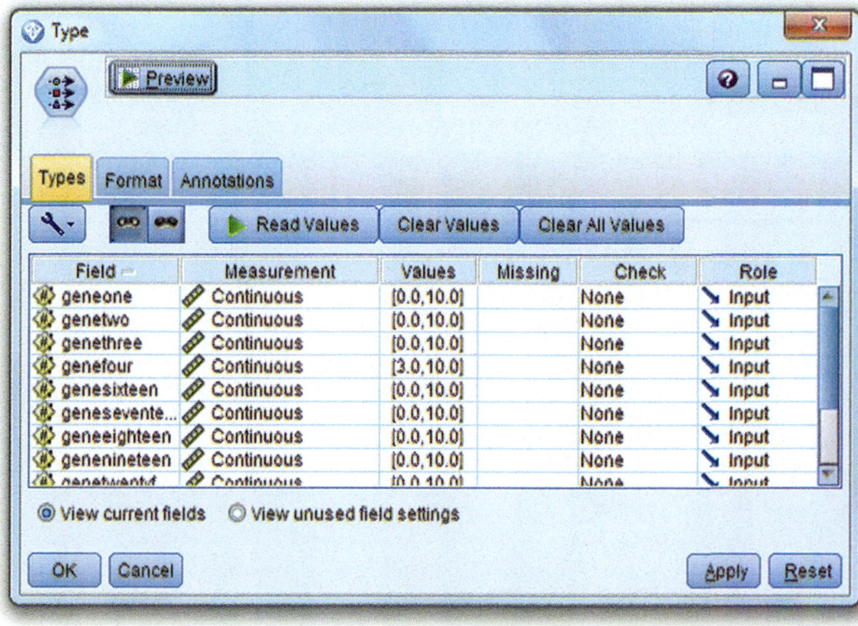

18.4.4 Step 4 the Auto Numeric Node

Now, click the Auto Numeric node and drag to canvas and connect with the Type node using the above connect-procedure. Click the Auto Numeric node, and the underneath graph comes up.…now click Model.…select Correlation as metric to rank quality of the various analysis methods used.… the additional manoeuvres are as indicated below.…in Numbers of models to use: type the number 3.

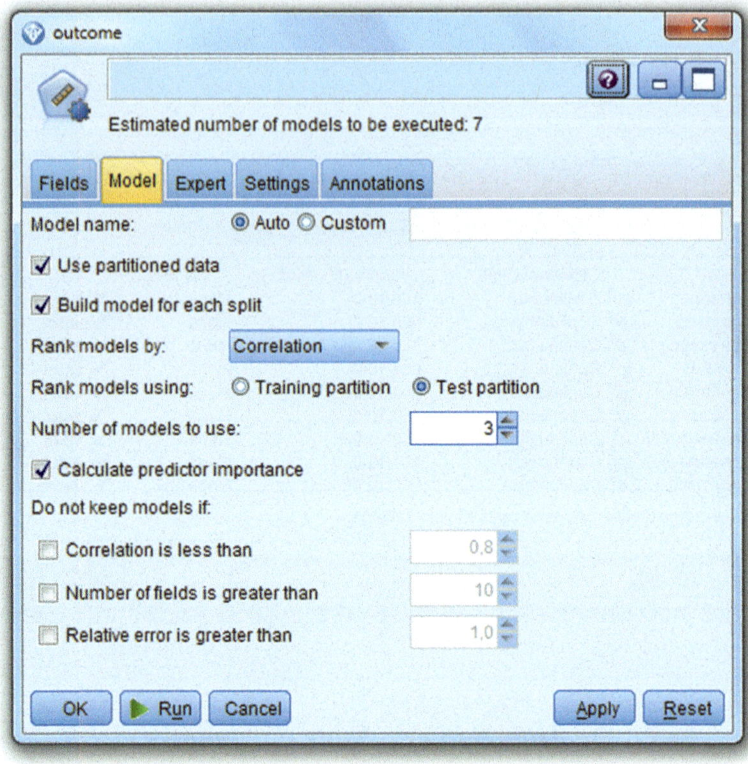

18.4.5 Step 5 the Expert Node

Then click the Expert tab. It is shown below. Out of 7 statistical models the three best fit ones are used by SPSS modeler for the ensembled model.

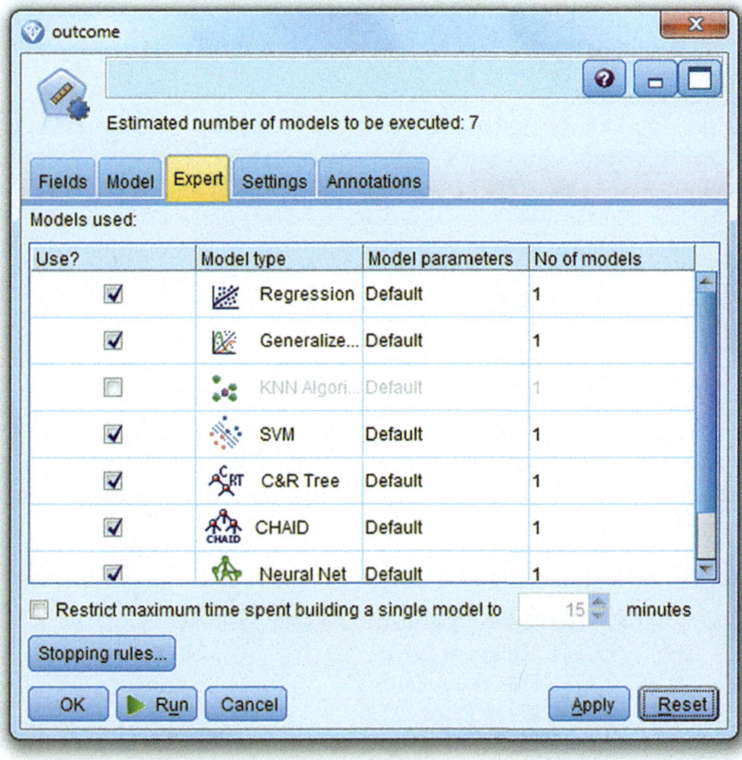

The 7 statistical models include:

1/. Linear regression (Regression)
2/. Generalized linear model (Generalized. . . .)
3/. K nearest neighbor clustering (KNN Algorithm)
4/. Support vector machine (SVM)
5/. Classification and regression tree (C&R Tree)
6/. Chi square automatic interaction detection (CHAID Tree)
7/. Neural network (Neural Net)

18.4.6 Step 6 the Settings Tab

In the underneath graph click the Settings tab. . . .click the Run button. . . .now a gold nugget is placed on the canvas. . . .click the gold nugget. . . .the model created is shown below.

Use?	Graph	Model	Build Time (mins)	Correlation	No. Fields Used	Relative Error
✓		CHAID 1	< 1	0,854	8	0,271
✓		SVM 1	< 1	0,836	12	0,304
✓		Regressi...	< 1	0,821	12	0,326

The correlation coefficients of the three best models are over 0.8, and, thus, pretty good. We will now perform the ensembled procedure.

18.4.7 Step 7 the Analysis Node

Find in the palettes below the screen the Analysis node and drag it to the canvas. With the above connect procedure connect it with the gold nugget....click the Analysis node.

Comparing $XR-outcome with outcome

Minimum Error	-2,878
Maximum Error	3,863
Mean Error	-0,014
Mean Absolute Error	0,77
Standard Deviation	1,016
Linear Correlation	0,859
Occurrences	250

The above table is shown and gives the statistics of the ensembled model created. The ensembled outcome is the average score of the scores from the three best fit statistical models. Adjustment for multiple testing and for variance stabilization with Fisher transformation is automatically carried out. The ensembled outcome (named the $XR-outcome) is compared with the outcomes of the three best fit statistical models, namely, CHAID (chi square automatic interaction detector), SVM (support vector machine), and Regression (linear regression). The ensembled correlation coefficient is larger (0.859) than the correlation coefficients from the three best fit models (0.854, 0.836, 0.821), and, so, ensembled procedures make sense, because they can provide increased precision in the analysis. The ensembled model can now be stored as an SPSS Modeler Stream file for future use in the appropriate folder of your computer. For the readers' convenience it is in extras.springer.com, and it is entitled "ensembledmodelcontinuous".

In the example given in this chapter, the ensembled correlation coefficient is larger (0.859) than the correlation coefficients from the three best fit models (0.854, 0.836, 0.821), and, so, ensembled procedures do make sense, because they can provide increased precision in the analysis.

18.5 Discussion

Automatic modeling of continuous outcomes computes the ensembled result of a number of best fit models for a particular data set, and provides better sensitivity of testing than the separate analysis models do. This chapter assessed, whether it can be used for efficacy analysis of clinical trials, and to test its performance against that of traditional efficacy analysis for the purpose. The traditional analysis showed that all of the genes were very significant predictors. In order to adjust confounding multiple regressions were performed. Six out of twelve genes were significant, and after Bonferroni adjustment only four out of twelve remained so. The ensembled procedures gave from the three best fit machine learning models out of seven the correlation coefficients:

Chi-square Automatic Interaction Detection	R	=	0.854
Support Vector Machines	R	=	0.836
Linear Regression	R	=	0.821

The pooled correlation coefficient from the above three was 0.859. We conclude that the ensembled procedure provides valuable information additional to that of the traditional efficacy analysis.

In this chapter the traditional efficacy analysis consisted of simple linear regressions, multiple linear regressions, and Bonferroni's adjustments, and the machine learning analyses included ensembled correlation models. The machine learning analyses provided better sensitivity of testing, and were more informative.

18.6 References

To readers requesting more background, theoretical and mathematical information of computations given, several textbooks complementary to the current production and also written by the same authors are available:

Statistics applied to clinical studies 5th edition, 2012,
Machine learning in medicine a complete overview, 2015,
SPSS for starters and 2nd levelers 2nd edition, 2015,
Clinical data analysis on a pocket calculator 2nd edition, 2016,
Understanding clinical data analysis from published research, 2016,
Modern meta-analysis, 2017,
Regression analysis in clinical research, 2018,
Modern Bayesian statistics in clinical research, 2018.
The analysis of safety data of drug trials an update, 2019.

All of them have been edited by Springer Heidelberg Germany.

Chapter 19
Gamma-Distributions for Efficacy Analysis

Contents

Abstract In a 110 patient random sample, the effects of age, psychological, and social scores on health scores were tested, both traditionally, and with the help of machine learning.

Traditional efficacy analysis consisted of

simple linear regressions,
multiple linear regressions,
Bonferroni's adjustments.

Machine learning efficacy analysis consisted of gamma-distribution methods.

The machine learning methods provided better sensitivity of testing, and were more informative.

Keywords Clinical trials · Traditional efficacy analysis · Machine learning efficacy analysis · Gamma-distribution methods

19.1 Introduction

Factors like age classes, psychological scores, and social scores are like treatment modalities of an interventional drug trial. Better drugs predict better health outcomes. And so do better age classes and better psychological scores predict better levels of health or disease. Traditionally, chi-square tests are applied for discrete predictors and discrete outcomes, while linear regressions are applied for continuous (or discrete) predictors and continuous outcomes are applied. The gamma

T. J. Cleophas, A. H. Zwinderman, *Efficacy Analysis in Clinical Trials an Update*,
https://doi.org/10.1007/978-3-030-19918-0_19

frequency distribution is suitable for statistical testing of nonnegative data with a continuous outcome variable, and fits such data often better than does the normal frequency distribution, particularly when magnitudes of benefits or risks is the outcome, like costs.

By readers not fond of maths the next few lines can be skipped.

The gamma frequency distribution ranges, like the Poisson distribution for rate assessments, from 0-∞. It is bell-shaped, like the normal distribution, but not as symmetric, looking a little like the chi-square distribution. Its algebraic approximation resembles is given underneath.

$$y = e^\wedge - 1/2\ x^2 \text{ (standardized normal distribution)}$$

$$y = (\lambda x)^r/\gamma * e^\wedge - \lambda x \text{ (gamma distribution)}$$

where
λ = scale parameter
r = shape parameter
γ = correction constant
^ = symbol of exponential term that follows.

This chapter is to assess, whether gamma distributions are also helpful for the efficacy analysis of medical data, particularly those with outcome scores. We will test traditional efficacy analysis against gamma analysis as computationally intensive machine learning methodology. Traditional efficacy analysis will consist of simple linear regressions, multiple linear regressions, and Bonferroni's adjustments.

19.2 Data Example

In 110 patients the effects of age, psychological and social score on health scores was assessed. The first 10 patients are underneath. The entire data file is entitled "gamma", and is in extras.springer.com.

age	psychologic score	social score	health score
3	5	4	8
1	4	8	7
1	5	13	4
1	4	15	6
1	7	4	10
1	8	8	6
1	9	12	8
1	8	16	2
1	12	4	6
1	13	1	8

age = age class 1-7
psychologicscore = psychological score 1-20
socialscore = social score 1-20
healthscore = health score 1-20.

Start by opening the data file in your computer mounted with SPSS statistical software. We will first perform a traditional efficacy analysis with linear regressions.

19.3 Traditional Efficacy Analysis

Traditional efficacy analysis consists of t-tests for continuous outcomes and chi-square tests for discrete outcomes. In Sect. 1.12, Chap. 1, the use of regression analyses for efficacy analyses is discussed, and in Sect. 1.13 the use of clinical trials for the assessment of causal health effects of factors other than medicines is discussed. For example, effects of interventions like angioplasties, surgeries, renal transplants etc. Many more factors can be tested in clinical trials, for example,

age factors
psychological factors
social factors
physical factors
economical factors,
and, any factor with a supposedly causal effect on health or sickness.

Start by opening the data file in your computer mounted with SPSS statistical software. We will now perform linear regressions.

Command

Analyze....Regression....Linear....Dependent: enter healthscore....Independent (s): enter socialscore....click OK.

The underneath table gives the result. Social score seems to be a very significant predictor of health score.

Coefficients[a]

Model		Unstandardized Coefficients		Standardized Coefficients	t	Sig.
		B	Std. Error	Beta		
1	(Constant)	9.833	.535		18.388	.000
	social score	-.334	.050	-.541	-6.690	.000

a. Dependent Variable: health score

Similarly psychological score and age class are tested.

Coefficients[a]

Model		Unstandardized Coefficients		Standardized Coefficients	t	Sig.
		B	Std. Error	Beta		
1	(Constant)	5.152	.607		8.484	.000
	psychological score	.140	.054	.241	2.575	.011

a. Dependent Variable: health score

Coefficients[a]

Model		Unstandardized Coefficients		Standardized Coefficients	t	Sig.
		B	Std. Error	Beta		
1	(Constant)	7.162	.588		12.183	.000
	age class	-.149	.133	-.107	-1.118	.266

a. Dependent Variable: health score

Three univariate linear regressions with the predictors as independent variables and health scores as outcome suggests, that both psychological and social scores are significant predictors of health, but age is not. In order to assess confounding, a multiple linear regression will be performed.

Command

Analyze. . . .Regression. . . .Linear. . . .Dependent: enter healthscore. . . .Independent (s): enter socialscore, psychologicscore, age. . . .click OK.

Coefficients[a]

Model		Unstandardized Coefficients		Standardized Coefficients	t	Sig.
		B	Std. Error	Beta		
1	(Constant)	9.388	.870		10.788	.000
	social score	-.329	.049	-.533	-6.764	.000
	psychological score	.111	.046	.190	2.418	.017
	age class	-.184	.109	-.132	-1.681	.096

a. Dependent Variable: health score

The above table is in the output. Social score is again very significant. Psychological score also, but after Bonferroni adjustment (rejection p-value = 0.05/4 = 0.0125) it would be no more so, because p = 0.017 is larger than 0.0125. Age is again not significant. Health score is here a continuous variable of nonnegative values, and perhaps a better fit of these data could be obtained by a gamma regression. We will use SPSS statistical software again.

19.4 Gamma-Distributions for Efficacy Analysis

Command

Analyze....click Generalized Linear Models....click once again Generalized Linear Models....mark Custom....Distribution: select Gamma....Link function: select Power....Power: type -1....click Response....Dependent Variable: enter healthscore click Predictors....Factors: enter socialscore, psychologicscore, age ....Model: enter socialscore, psychologicscore, age....Estimation: Scale Parameter Method: select Pearson chi-square....click EM Means: Displays Means for: enter age, psychologicscore, socialscore....click Save....mark Predict value of linear predictor....Standardize deviance residual....click OK.

Tests of Model Effects

Source	Type III		
	Wald Chi-Square	df	Sig.
(Intercept)	216.725	1	.000
ageclass	8.838	6	.183
psychologicscore	18.542	13	.138
socialscore	61.207	13	.000

Dependent Variable: health score
Model: (Intercept), ageclass, psychologicscore, socialscore

The above table gives the overall result: it is similar to that of the traditional multiple linear regression with only social class as significant independent predictor.

However, also in the output are shown additional tables: gamma regression tables to test various levels of predictive strength of the separate predictors.

Parameter Estimates

Parameter	B	Std. Error	95% Wald Confidence Interval		Hypothesis Test		
			Lower	Upper	Wald Chi-Square	df	Sig.
(Intercept)	.188	.0796	.032	.344	5.566	1	.018
[ageclass=1]	-.017	.0166	-.050	.015	1.105	1	.293
[ageclass=2]	-.002	.0175	-.036	.032	.010	1	.919
[ageclass=3]	-.015	.0162	-.047	.017	.839	1	.360
[ageclass=4]	.014	.0176	-.020	.049	.658	1	.417
[ageclass=5]	.025	.0190	-.012	.062	1.723	1	.189
[ageclass=6]	.005	.0173	-.029	.039	.087	1	.767
[ageclass=7]	0[a]	.	.	.	.	.	.
[psychologicscore=3]	.057	.0409	-.023	.137	1.930	1	.165
[psychologicscore=4]	.057	.0220	.014	.100	6.754	1	.009
[psychologicscore=5]	.066	.0263	.015	.118	6.352	1	.012
[psychologicscore=7]	.060	.0311	-.001	.121	3.684	1	.055
[psychologicscore=8]	.061	.0213	.019	.102	8.119	1	.004
[psychologicscore=9]	.035	.0301	-.024	.094	1.381	1	.240
[psychologicscore=11]	.057	.0325	-.007	.120	3.059	1	.080
[psychologicscore=12]	.060	.0219	.017	.103	7.492	1	.006
[psychologicscore=13]	.040	.0266	-.012	.092	2.267	1	.132
[psychologicscore=14]	.090	.0986	-.103	.283	.835	1	.361
[psychologicscore=15]	.121	.0639	-.004	.247	3.610	1	.057
[psychologicscore=16]	.041	.0212	-.001	.082	3.698	1	.054
[psychologicscore=17]	.022	.0241	-.025	.069	.841	1	.359
[psychologicscore=18]	0[a]	.	.	.	.	.	.
[socialscore=4]	-.120	.0761	-.269	.029	2.492	1	.114
[socialscore=6]	-.028	.0986	-.221	.165	.079	1	.778
[socialscore=8]	-.100	.0761	-.249	.050	1.712	1	.191
[socialscore=9]	.002	.1076	-.209	.213	.000	1	.988
[socialscore=10]	-.123	.0864	-.293	.046	2.042	1	.153
[socialscore=11]	.015	.0870	-.156	.185	.029	1	.865
[socialscore=12]	-.064	.0772	-.215	.088	.682	1	.409
[socialscore=13]	-.065	.0773	-.216	.087	.703	1	.402
[socialscore=14]	.008	.0875	-.163	.180	.009	1	.925
[socialscore=15]	-.051	.0793	-.207	.104	.420	1	.517
[socialscore=16]	.026	.0796	-.130	.182	.107	1	.744
[socialscore=17]	-.109	.0862	-.277	.060	1.587	1	.208
[socialscore=18]	-.053	.0986	-.246	.141	.285	1	.593
[socialscore=19]	0[a]	.	.	.	.	.	.
(Scale)	.088[b]						

Dependent Variable: health score
Model: (Intercept), ageclass, psychologicscore, socialscore

a. Set to zero because this parameter is redundant.
b. Computed based on the Pearson chi-square.

As shown in the above large table, gamma regression enables to test various regression coefficients (b values) of the predictor scores separately. Age classes were not significant predictors. Of the psychological scores, however, no less than 8 scores produced pretty small p-values, even as small as 0.004–0.009. Of the social scores now no score is significant

. In order to better understand, what is going on, SPSS provides a marginal means analysis here.

Estimates

age class	Mean	Std. Error	95% Wald Confidence Interval	
			Lower	Upper
1	5.62	.531	4.58	6.66
2	5.17	.461	4.27	6.07
3	5.54	.489	4.59	6.50
4	4.77	.402	3.98	5.56
5	4.54	.391	3.78	5.31
6	4.99	.439	4.13	5.85
7	5.12	.453	4.23	6.01

The mean health outcome scores of the different age classes were, indeed, hardly different.

Estimates

psychological score	Mean	Std. Error	95% Wald Confidence Interval	
			Lower	Upper
3	5.03	.997	3.08	6.99
4	5.02	.404	4.23	5.81
5	4.80	.541	3.74	5.86
7	4.96	.695	3.60	6.32
8	4.94	.359	4.23	5.64
9	5.64	.809	4.05	7.22
11	5.03	.752	3.56	6.51
12	4.95	.435	4.10	5.81
13	5.49	.586	4.34	6.64
14	4.31	1.752	.88	7.74
15	3.80	.898	2.04	5.56
16	5.48	.493	4.51	6.44
17	6.10	.681	4.76	7.43
18	7.05	1.075	4.94	9.15

However, increasing psychological scores seem to be associated with increasing levels of health outcome.

Estimates

social score	Mean	Std. Error	95% Wald Confidence Interval	
			Lower	Upper
4	8.07	.789	6.52	9.62
6	4.63	1.345	1.99	7.26
8	6.93	.606	5.74	8.11
9	4.07	1.266	1.59	6.55
10	8.29	2.838	2.73	13.86
11	3.87	.634	2.62	5.11
12	5.55	.529	4.51	6.59
13	5.58	.558	4.49	6.68
14	3.96	.711	2.57	5.36
15	5.19	.707	3.81	6.58
16	3.70	.371	2.98	4.43
17	7.39	2.256	2.96	11.81
18	5.23	1.616	2.06	8.40
19	4.10	1.280	1.59	6.61

In contrast, increasing social scores are, obviously, associated with decreasing levels of health outcome, with mean health scores sometimes close to 3 in the higher social score patients, and close to 10 in the lower social score patients.

19.5 Discussion

Factors like age classes, psychological scores, and social scores are like treatment modalities of an interventional drug trial. Better drugs predict better health outcomes. And so may higher age classes and higher psychological scores predict higher levels of health or disease. Traditionally, chi-square tests and linear regressions are applied for efficacy analyses. The gamma frequency distribution is, however, very suitable for statistical testing of nonnegative data with a continuous outcome variable, and fits such data better than does the normal frequency distribution, particularly when magnitudes of benefits or risks is in the outcome. The example given shows, that gamma regression is a worthwhile analysis model complementary to linear regression, and that it elucidates effects unobserved in the traditional models.

In this chapter the traditional efficacy analysis consisted of simple linear regressions, multiple linear regressions, and Bonferroni's adjustments, and the machine learning analyses included gamma distribution models. The machine learning analyses provided better sensitivity of testing, and were more informative.

19.6 References

To readers requesting more background, theoretical and mathematical information of computations given, several textbooks complementary to the current production and written by the same authors are available:

Statistics applied to clinical studies 5th edition, 2012,
Machine learning in medicine a complete overview, 2015,
SPSS for starters and 2nd levelers 2nd edition, 2015,
Clinical data analysis on a pocket calculator 2nd edition, 2016,
Understanding clinical data analysis from published research, 2016,
Modern meta-analysis, 2017,
Regression analysis in clinical research, 2018,
Modern Bayesian statistics in clinical research, 2018.
The Analysis of Safety Data of Drug Trials, an Update, 2019.

All of them have been edited by Springer Heidelberg Germany.

Chapter 20
Validating Big Data, a Big Issue

Contents

Abstract Big data consist of multiple fractions of small data. If you wish your big data to be valid, then you will, first, have to make sure, that the fractions are validated:

by the use of the scientific rules for clinical trials, and, in addition,

by the use of traditional diagnostic test validations.

Once this is all done well and good, only then you will be at the starting point of a serious big data analysis. Unfortunately, this is a pretty laborious scenario, and, although, currently, many data bases of big data do exist, most of them are, documentedly, of a poor quality and un-validated. Big data analyses tend to suffer from too many null-values, lack of experienced analysis teams, lacking validation tools, limited validation checklists. Big data tools are in expensive commercial software, and have not been judged by Academia. The best approach to big data analyses may be the use of large checklists, multiple analysis teams, and the use of multiple independent computers with simple programs rather than supercomputers with complex programs.

Keywords Big data validation · Clinical trial validation · Scientific rules for clinical trials · Diagnostic test validation

T. J. Cleophas, A. H. Zwinderman, *Efficacy Analysis in Clinical Trials an Update*,
https://doi.org/10.1007/978-3-030-19918-0_20

20.1 Introduction

Validation may be a semantic term. Yet validation is the most important part of big data studies, and, currently, demands more than half of the time spent on big data analysis (Xie C, Big data validation case study. Published by IEEE Computer Society, 2017, Doi 10.1109 BigDataService). In clinical research the term validation refers, according to the American FDA (Process Validation Doc 2016), to process design, process qualification, continuous process verification, and different types are implicated, like retrospective, prospective, concurrent validation, and re-validation. With diagnostic tests, which are commonly called the basis of clinical research, validation consists of accuracy, reproducibility, precision assessments (Statistics applied to clinical studies 5th edition, from the same authors, Springer Heidelberg Germany, 2012). With clinical trial protocols validation consists of a clearly defined prior hypothesis, a valid design, explicit description of methods, and uniform data analysis.

Validating big data can, theoretically, be accomplished using all of the rules applied with small data, but this is very laborious, if not hardly possible. If big data consists of a pool of multiple small data, special checks are required, like publication bias, heterogeneity, robustness checks. Tentative alternatives for big data validation are occasionally given. In the above reference from Xie it says: multiple teams are appointed to validate fractions of data analyses. In the Hadoop framework 2014, an interesting open-source framework to process and store big data (www.tutorialspoint.com), multiple standard computers with multiple relatively simple programs are advisedly applied for accomplishing big data validations. The current chapter will summarize traditional validation tools for relatively small data, and, in addition, refer to important tentative tools especially designed for big data validation.

20.2 Semantics of the Term Validation

In Google's Your Dictionary examples are given of semantics. For example, a water pill is a pill filled with water. However, to others it is a diuretic. Or the term crash has multiple meanings: car accident, drop of stocks, attending a party without being invited, ocean waves hitting the shore, sound of cymbals being struck together. The term validation is another semantic one: according to the Cambridge English Dictionary, it is:

(1) the action of checking or proving the validity or accuracy of something, for example in "the technique requires validation in controlled trials",
(2) the action of making or declaring something legally or officially acceptable, for example in "new courses, subject to validation, include an MSc in Urban Forestry",

(3) recognition or affirmation that a person or their feelings or opinions are valid or worthwhile, for example in “they have exaggerated needs for acceptance and validations”.

With Drug Manufacturing it means (according to the GMP (good manufacturing practice) guidelines enforced by the American Food and drug administration (FDA): Validation is the process of establishing documentary evidence, meanwhile demonstrating that a procedure, process, or activity is carried out in testing, and then production maintains the desired level of compliance at all stages.

According to the FDA (Process Validation Doc 2016): three stages are implicated:

1. Process design
2. Process qualification
3. Continued process verification

And four types are implicated:

1. Retrospective validation
2. Prospective validation
3. Concurrent Validation
4. Revalidation.

20.3 Clinical Trial Validation

In the year 2000 the title “Statistics applied to clinical trials” now in its 5th edition and from the same authors was published by Springer Heidelberg Germany. Validation is the most important part of clinical trials. In the first lines of the title an effort was given to summarize the validation process.

A. *Clearly defined hypotheses*
   Hypotheses must be tested prospectively with hard data, and against placebo or known forms of therapies that are in place and considered to be effective. Uncontrolled studies won’t succeed to give a definitive answer if they are ever so clever. Uncontrolled studies while of value in the absence of scientific controlled studies, their conclusions represent merely suggestions and hypotheses. The scientific method requires to look at some controls to characterize the defined population.
B. *Valid designs*
   Any research but certainly industrially sponsored drug research where sponsors benefit from favorable results, benefits from valid designs. A valid study means a study unlikely to be biased, or unlikely to include systematic errors. The most dangerous errors in clinical trials are systematic errors otherwise called biases. Validity is the most important thing for doers of clinical trials to check. Trials should be made independent, objective, balanced, blinded, controlled, with objective measurements, with adequate sample sizes to test the expected treatment effects, with random assignment of patients.

C. *Explicit description of methods*
Explicit description of the methods should include description of the recruitment procedures, method of randomization of the patients, prior statements about the methods of assessments of generating and analysis of the data and the statistical methods used, accurate ethics including written informed consent.

D. *Uniform data analysis*
Uniform and appropriate data analysis generally starts with plots or tables of actual data. Statistics then comes in to test primary hypotheses primarily. Data that do not answer prior hypotheses may be tested for robustness or sensitivity, otherwise called precision of point estimates e.g., dependent upon numbers of outliers. The results of studies with many outliers and thus little precision should be interpreted with caution. It is common practice for studies to test multiple measurements for the purpose of answering one single question. In clinical trials the benefit to health is estimated by variables, which can be defined as measurable factors or characteristics used to estimate morbidity/mortality/time to events etc. Variables are named exposure, indicator, or independent variables, if they predict morbidity/mortality, and outcome or dependent variables, if they estimate morbidity/mortality. Sometimes both mortality and morbidity variables are used in a single trial, and there is nothing wrong with that practice. We should not make any formal correction for multiple comparisons of this kind of data. Instead, we should informally integrate all the data before reaching conclusions, and look for the trends without judging one or two low P-values among otherwise high P-values as proof.

Clinical trials are different from big data, but a type of research, which looks a bit like big data, is the method of systematic review of clinical trials, and, if complemented with a statistical work-up, the method of meta-analysis. The above validation process was used again in the authors' title of 2017 "Modern meta-analysis", also edited by Springer. Like with clinical trials, the most important part of meta-analyses is validation. The title's first chapter entitled "Meta-analysis in a nutshell" addressed the four points already applied with clinical trial validation, although with slightly different terminology.

> All that is needed for a (read: valid) meta-analysis, is the rules of scientific rigor and a brief list of pitfalls is given. Scientific rigor requires that we stick to
>
> (1) a clearly defined prior hypothesis,
> (2) a thorough search of trials,
> (3) strict inclusion criteria,
> (4) uniform guidelines for data analysis.
>
> A brief list of pitfalls includes
>
> (1) checking publication bias,
> (2) checking heterogeneity,
> (3) checking robustness.

Validation does not only include quality criteria for clinical trial validations, but also quality criteria for diagnostic tests. Not the trials, but rather the diagnostic tests are the heart of evidence-based medicine. The STARD (Standards for reporting diagnostic accuracy) group launched in 2003 quality criteria for diagnostic tests, and updated them in 2015 (Bossuyt et al., BMJ 2015; 351: h5527).

Apart from 25 very general topics addressed, the topics 12 and 13 covered the subject statistical methods, which we will cite:

12. Methods for calculating and comparing measures of diagnostic accuracy, and the statistical methods used to quantify uncertainty (e.g. 95% confidence intervals).
13. Methods for calculating test reproducibility, if done.

Unfortunately, the STARD group guidelines are very liberate, and they never addressed specific methods and/or specific tests to be performed, and, thus, are not very helpful to eliminate the underneath flawed methods and incorrect tests.

20.4 Diagnostic Test Validation

Diagnostic tests must be valid. The term valid sensu stricto does include the following.

1. Valid = accurate.
2. Reproducible = reliable.
3. Precise = with a small spread.

Intervention trials may be well paid, published in high impact journal, and the may provide excellent career perspectives. In contrast, evaluations of diagnostic tests are not well paid, difficult to publish, they provide a poor career perspective, and the are often (post or propter) performed in sloppy ways. Yet intervention trials are impossible without diagnostic tests. We might say, diagnostic tests is the only real basis of evidence-based medicine. Young investigators are often requested to test diagnostic tests. How to do so?

1. Assess validity, i.e., the test shows who has the disease, and who has not.
2. Assess reproducibility, i.e., the second test produced the same result.
3. Assess precision, i.e., a small spread is in the data.

Diagnostic tests are, traditionally, classified.

(1) qualitative (the "yes/no" tests or binary tests).

An example is "an elevated erythrocyte sedimentation rate above 32 mm for diagnosis of pneumonia".

(2) quantitative (outcome values have a continuous character).

An example is "the echographical cardiac output measurements around 5 liter/min".

A table of methods for assessing validated, otherwise called high quality, diagnostic tests is given underneath.

	validity	reproducibility	precision
Qualitative tests	sensitivity specificity overall validity ROC curves	Cohen's kappas	SDs, SEs 95% ci
Quantitative tests	linear regression (test a = 0, b = 1) paired t-test Bland-Altman plot complex regressions	duplicate SD repeatability coefficient intraclass correlation	SDs, SEs 95% ci data modeling

ROC = receiver operating characteristic, SD = standard deviation, SE = standard error, a = intercept of linear regression, b = regression coefficient of linear regression

Statistics is for Providing Quality Criteria for Diagnostic Tests, Validity, Reproducibility, and Precision of Qualitative Tests.

1. Validity of Qualitative Tests

The underneath table shows healthy and unhealthy subjects. The b and c subjects are false negative and false positive respectively. They are the problem of diagnostics tests.

Disease	yes (n)	no (n)
Positive test	a	b
Negative test	c	d

a = number of true positive patients
b = false positive patients
c = false negative patients
d = true negative patients

Sensitivity = a / (a + c) = (false positives) / (false positive + false negatives)
Specificity = d / (b + d) = (true negatives) / (true negatives + false positives)
Overall validity = (a + d) / (a + b + c + d)

Example. Patients are assessed for pneumonia consist of 2 Gaussian groups: on x-axis individ ESRs, y-axis how often. Various "normal values" can be considered .

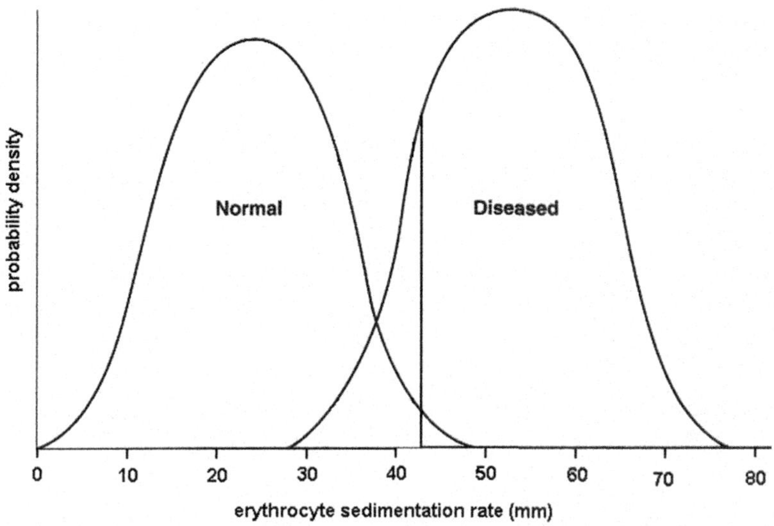

If the "normal value" is an ESR (erythrocyte sedimentation rate) of 43 mm, then, according to the test, right from 43 mm the patients are diseased. You will miss many diseaseds. This test would have a low sensitivity. Your beta would be large, and your alpha would be small.

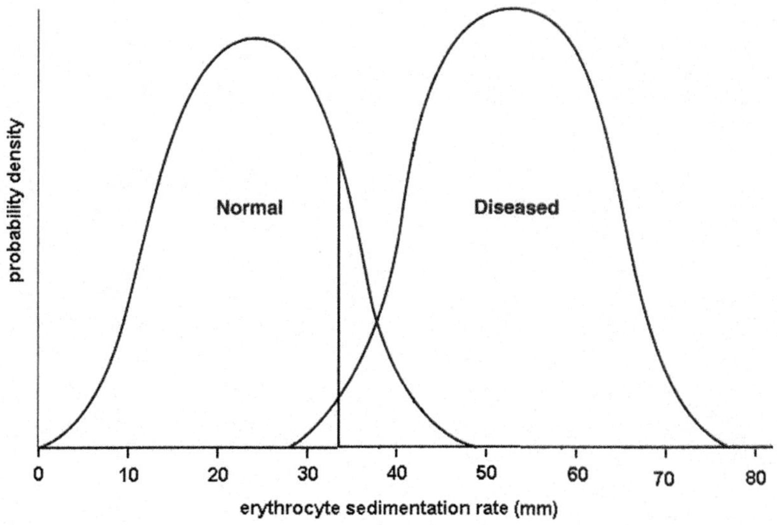

If the ESR is 32 mm, then, according to the test, right from 32 mm the patients will be diseased. You miss many healthy patients. The test has a low specificity. Your beta will be small, and your alpha will be large.

(beta = type II error of finding no effect, where there is one, alpha = type I error of finding an effect, where there is none)

Now, what cut-off value or "normal" value is best? You want to miss few diagnoses, thus, wish to have a high sensitivity and specificity. ROC (receiver operating characteristic) curves are helpful for finding out. Calculate for several normal-values the corresponding sensitivities and specificities. Then draw a curve with on the y-axis sensitivities, and on the x-axis specificities or, rather, (1-specificities) = proportion of false positives. A perfect diagnostic test will reach the top y-axis (100% sensitivity, 100% specificity), but, unfortunately, this will never happen.

In the underneath graph an example is given. With an ESR (erythrocyte sedimentation rate) of 38 mm the shortest distance to the top of the y-axis is obtained.

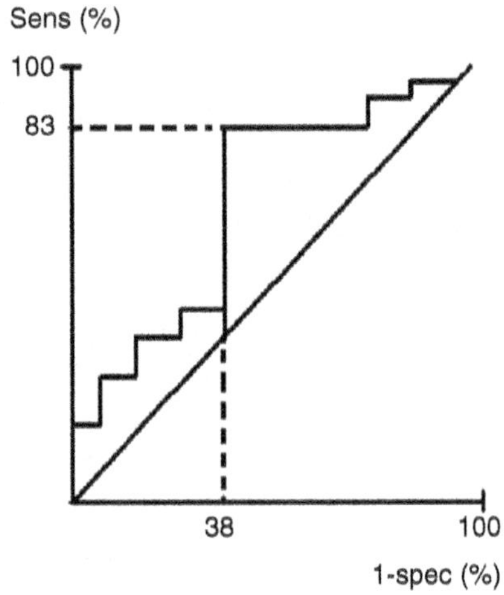

ROC curves are very popular but....

1. Sometimes more than a single shortest distance from the top of the y-axis is observed.
2. A curve close to the diagonal may exist and indicates a poor test, because sensitivity and specificity together will never exceed approximately 100%, e.g., 45% and 55%, a sensitivity or specificity close to 50% is a result similar to that of gambling, like tossing a coin. Such a test is poor, because it can be replaced with gambling.
3. Comparing 2 curves for finding the best of 2 diagnostic tests is called c-statistics. The problem is that the curves often cross with intervals where one test performs better than the other vice versa.

2. Reproducibility of Qualitative Tests

Cohen's kappas are, traditionally, used for assessing the reproducibility or reliability of a qualitative diagnostic test. An example is given. A lab-test includes 30 patients. All patients are tested twice.

		1st time		
		yes	no	
2nd time	yes	10	5	15
	no	4	11	15
	14	16	30	

If not reproducible at all, you should find 15 × twice the same (half of the times the same outcome. We do, however, find 21 × twice the same.

$$\text{Kappa} = \frac{\text{observed - minimal}}{\text{maximal - minimal}} = \frac{21\text{-}15}{30\text{-}15} = 0.4$$

A result of 0.4 is better than not reproducible at all, 0 means very poor, 1 excellent reliability.

3. Precision of Qualitative Tests

In order to assess the precision of your qualitative diagnostic test, calculate measures of spread in your outcome data, e.g., SEs (standard errors) or 95% confidence intervals (± 2SEMS). The SEs of the sensitivity and specificity are calculated as follows.

Sensitivity (if sens = a/(a + c), then its SE = $\sqrt{}$ [ac/(a + c)^3].

Specificity (if spec = d/(b + d),……

As an alternative, the underneath procedure is adequate. If 95% ci intervals cross a prior defined boundary, then the diagnostic test will not be valid (e.g., a boundary of 0.50 or 0.55 may be used). The STARD (standards for reporting diagnostic accuracy) Working Party (Section 8) says that precision of a qualitative diagnostic test is, traditionally, rarely assessed, and that, therefore, many tests, that are routinely used today, have been erroneously been validated in the past (see also Sect. 20.3 of this chapter).

We will now address the Validity, Reproducibility, and Precision of Quantitative Tests.

1. Validity of Quantitative Tests

The validity of quantitative tests are assessed with a special type of linear regression. An data example is given in the underneath graph.

On the x-axis (Variable 00002) we have echographical cardiac output.

On the y-axis (Variable 00001) we have an invasive measurement, the gold standard.

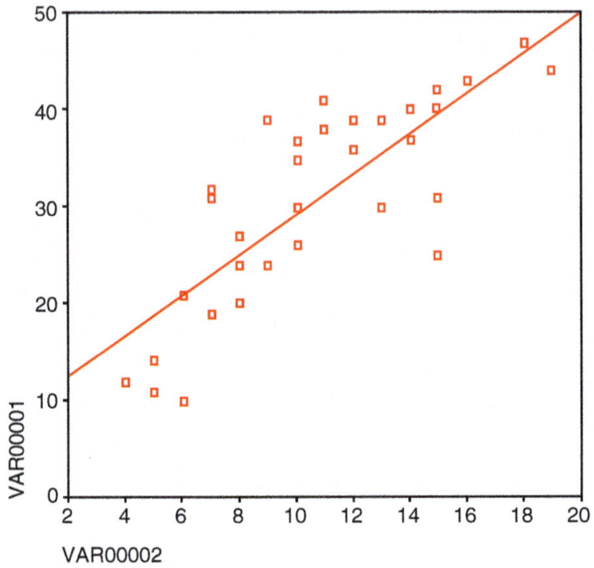

A significant correlation between the diagnostic test and the gold standard measurement is observed at $p < 0.0001$. However, the correlation coefficient with a p-value of good, but not good enough for approving, that this diagnostic test is valid.

Despite the small p-value, an enormous spread is in these data with huge departures from the best fit regression line. For example, if $x = 6$, then y would be close to 13 or 27. We will use the underneath procedure for validation purpose instead, and with better sensitivity:

Use the equation of regression line $y = a + bx$

a = intercept

b = direction coefficient

From the equation $y = a + bx$,

test if "a" is significantly different from 0, and

"b" is significantly different from 1.

If the 95% confidence interval of "b", being $2.065 \pm 2 \times 0.276$, contains 1.000, and.

"a", being $8.647 \pm 2 \times 3.132$, contains 0.000, only, then, validity will be accepted.

In the above example given:

"b" is between 1.513 and 2.617, and is, thus, > 1, and

"a" is between 2.383 and 14.911, and is, thus, > 0,

and, so, the diagnostic test is not valid.

Another data example is given. A new "mini" peakflow meter is validated, and is for that purpose compared to the standard peakflow meter. The underneath graph gives the validation data.

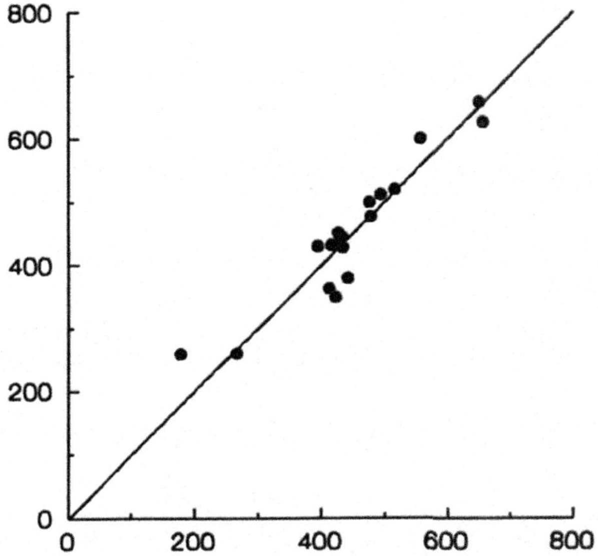

The 95% confidence interval of "b" = 0.917 ± 2 × 0.083 = between 0.751 and 1.083.

This interval contains the value 1.000.

The 95% confidence interval of "a" = 39.340 ± 2 × 38.704 = between −38.068 and 116.748.

This interval contains the value 0.000. The above diagnostic test is determined valid.

Additional methods for validating quantitative tests are widely used in the literature.

A few examples are given.

1. The paired t-test new diagnostic test versus the gold standard test (the difference should be not statistically significant)
2. The Bland-Altman plot uses the British Standards Institution repeatability coefficient: 95% of the paired differences should be within ± 2SDs (standard deviations).
3. Complex linear regression models can be used as well (e.g., Passing-Bablok and Deming regressions)

Two remarks should be made here.

1. The above three methods assume uncertainty of both the novel diagnostic test and the gold standard test. Generally, the latter of the two is not needed.
2. The above 2nd method does not account a sample size, and representative sample sizes are a requirement for validity assessments.

2. Reproducibility of Quantitative Tests

Many incorrect methods for assessing reproducibility of quantitative diagnostic tests are routinely used in research practice (Riegelman, Studying a study and testing a test, Lippincott Philadelphia PA, 2005). We are talking of popular sloppy-way methods.

1. A small mean difference between repeated tests.
2. A strong linear correlation between repeated tests.
3. Small coefficients of variation (= SD/mean × 100%), SD = standard deviation).

Examples of the above incorrect methods are given.

1st incorrect method: Calculate the means of the first and second set of tests. If the difference is small, then the diagnostic will be well reproducible.

test 1	test 2	difference
1	11	-10
10	0	10
2	11	-9
12	2	10
11	1	10
1	12	-11
mean difference		0

It is not hard to observe, that, despite the small difference between the means, the test is poorly reproducible, with a spread from −11 to +10.

2nd incorrect method: Draw a regression line with the test 1 results on x-axis, and the test 2 results on y- axis. If everything is close to the regression line, then the diagnostic test will be well reproducible.

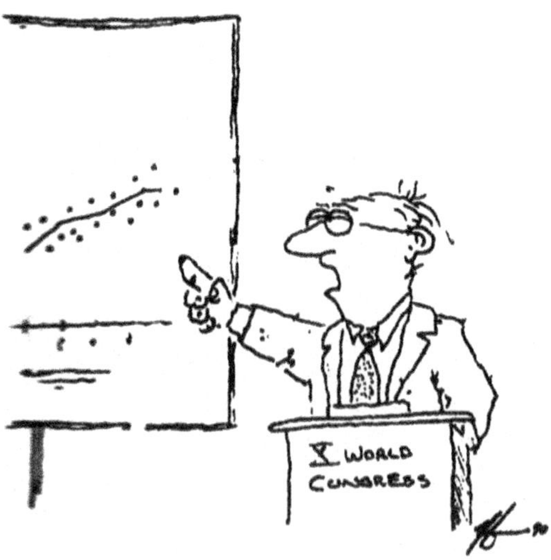

The diagnostic test is only reproducible, if the direction coefficient has a slope of 45°, and if the regression line crosses the x-axis through the basis of the y-axis.

3rd incorrect method: The coefficient of variation uses the eq. SD/mean × 100%. It does not account sample size, nor a second test.

The only correct methods for assessing reproducibility of quantitative diagnostic. tests are the three underneath.

1. Duplicate standard deviation (SD).
2. Repeatability coefficient.
3. Intraclass correlation.

Data examples are given.

1. Duplicate standard deviation

	test 1	test 2	difference(d)	$(\text{difference})^2$
	1	11	-10	100
	10	0	10	100
	2	11	-9	81
	12	2	10	100
	11	1	10	100
	1	12	-11	121
average	6.17	6.17	0	100.3

Duplicate SD = $\sqrt{(1/2 \times 100.3)} = 7.08$.
For accepting adequate reproducibility, it should be 10–20% of test-averages.

2. Repeatability coefficient

	test 1	test 2	difference
	1	11	- 10
	10	0	10
	2	11	- 9
	12	2	10
	11	1	10
	1	12	-11
Mean	6.17	6.17	

SD of differences = 10.97

Repeatability coefficient equals 2 SDs of the differences = 21.94
For accepting adequate reproducibility, it should be 10–20% of test-averages.

3. Intraclass correlation (ICC)

patient	test 1	test 2	SD^2
1	1	11	50
2	10	0	50
3	2	11	40.5
4	12	2	32
5	11	1	50
6	1	12	60.5
mean	6.17	6.17	

grand mean 6.17

SS between subjects = (mean test 1 – grand mean)^2 + (mean test 2 – grand mean)^2

SS between subjects = 0

SS within subjects = $SD_{patient1}{}^2 + SD_{.2}{}^2 + SD_{.3}{}^2 + SD_{.4}{}^2 + \ldots = 283$

$$ICC = \frac{\text{SS between subjects}}{\text{SS between subjects} + \text{SS within subjects}} = 0 - 1$$

If SS within = 0, then an excellent reproducibility is in the diagnostic test, because.

ICC = 1 (SS = sum of squares).

3. Precision of Quantitative Tests

A quantitative diagnostic test will be precise or robust, if the spread in data is small. Spread is usually assessed with standard deviations or standard errors. In situations, where reproducibility is poor, an increased precision can, usually, be obtained by data modeling. Examples are given.

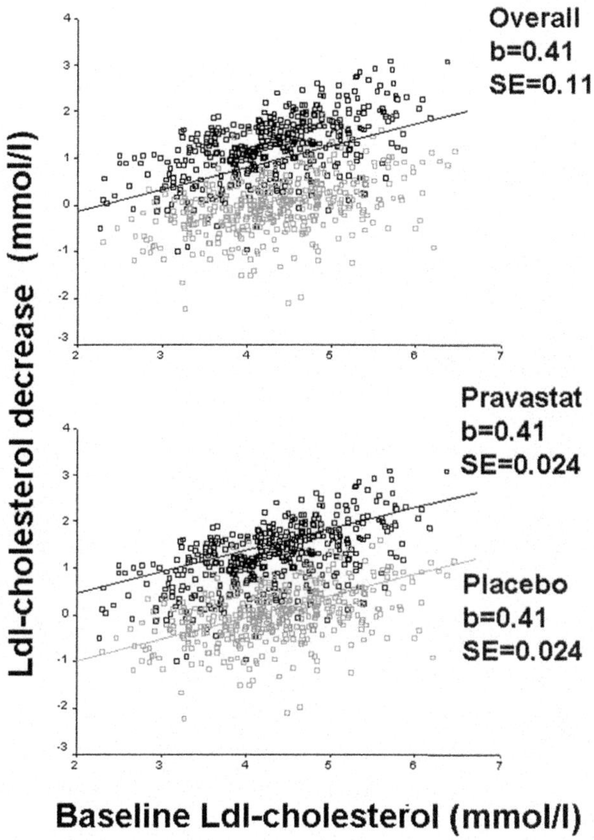

The above graph shows, that the spread of the data is pretty wide, with a standard error of 0.11 in the linear model. If, instead of a simple linear model, a two variables linear regression model is used with treatment modality as co-variable, the spread in the data reduces from a standard error (SE) of 0.11–0.024, which is much more precise.

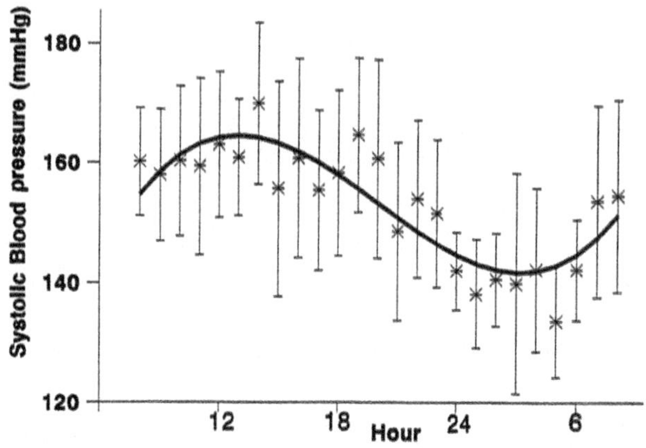

The above graph shows ambulatory blood pressure measurements. The spread of the data, as compared to the overall mean of the data, is assessed with the standard deviation. It equals 17 mm Hg. If, instead, the spread of the data is assessed with a curvilinear regression model, then it reduces from 17 to 7 mm Hg. The curvilinear model provides a much better precision for assessing these data, than the overall mean does.

20.5 Big Data Validation

Big data consist of multiple fractions of small data. If you wish your big data to be valid, then you will, first, have to make sure, that the fractions are validated as explained above:

by the use of the scientific rules for clinical trials, and, in addition,

by the use of the above diagnostic test validations.

Once this is all done well and good, only then you will be at the starting point of a serious big data analysis. Unfortunately, this is a pretty unrealistic scenario, and, although in the year 2018 many data bases of big data do exist, most of them are of a poor quality and un-validated, as shown in various case studies. (Gao et al. 2016; Woodall et al. 2015; Gassman et al. 1995; Laranjeiro et al. 2015; Becker et al. 2015)

In another recent case study from the computer engineering departments of San Jose University USA and Jiangsu University China, studying the results from an 8061-record case study of public weather data in California, the data were pretty simple. They only included sensor weather data. The results were, nonetheless, very disappointing. The findings:

1. too many null-values,
2. lack of trained teams,
3. lack of validation tools,
4. poor checks of consistency, compliance, missing data, data boundaries and ranges,
5. equally poor results of checks second to the above checks.

IEEE is an abbreviation of the Institute of Electrical and Electronic Engineers.

The IEEE Computer Society is the world's largest technical professional organization with its corporate office in New York City. In spite of the above disappointing results with big data analyses so far, the IEEE Computer Society has never stopped providing guidelines and recommendations.

Big data validation processes.

Process steps include:
1. data collection,
2. cleaning,
3. transformation,
4. validation sensu stricto
5. analysis and report

Big data quality checklist includes:

Different check lists are available for
1. Sensor data (17 checks)
2. Geospatial data (21 checks)
3. Health record data (16 checks)

Big data Tool Lists selected by IEEE include:

ETL (extraction transformation load program)
(UK)
Pentaho (from Hitachi) (Florida)
Tableau (visualization tool) (India)
Talend (multi-cloud integration and data-connection tool)
(Redwood California)
ZOHO (Indian software company, headquarter Chennai India).

The above validation tool lists must be operated by operation systems:

Operation Systems (OS) (Datameer)
Supported Files Systems (CVS, SPSS, Excel)
Supported Data Base Systems (Oracle, Windows).

Hadoop (2014) is an interesting open-source framework to store and process big data, and it uses instead of super computers clusters of normal computers using simple programming models. Hadoop's computers have two major layers, one for distribution computers, and one for storaging computers.

As shown above, checklists are pretty limited, and consist of only 17, 22, 16 checks, which is not many as compared to, for example, the double, triple, and counter checks routinely applied by airplane personnel before take off, which well amount to over 300 checks.

Many big data tools are commercial software, and very expensive, and have not been judged by Academia, and thus do not meet Academia standards.

No doubt one of the most proliferative type of big-data data files is the data files produced by high-tech technology companies. For example, Damen Shipyards Netherlands does monitor 150 vessels online, and does so with 6000 sensors per vessel with each sensor producing a datum per minute. The shipyard's offices are obviously snowed under with data. We should add, that all of the hundreds of thousands of sensors have been validated only once, in vitro at the office of the sensor building company, but they has never been validated on site. With the advent of big data, data is being generated, collected, transformed, processed and analyzed at an unprecedented scale. However, the quality of big data is far from perfect. Studies (Gao et al. 2016; Woodall et al. 2015; Gassman et al. 1995; Laranjeiro et al. 2015; Becker et al. 2015) have demonstrated that poor quality brings serious erroneous data and exorbitant data costs. Adequate data validation is the only possible way to recognize and improve poor quality data. The IEEE reports, that serious validation of big data currently consumes already over 50% of the time spent on big data projects. Big-data may be a hot research and application subject in academic research. The traditional principles of trial validations and data validations summarized in this chapter must play a principal role for the purpose of answering: what are the key factors to affect and improve big data quality, and to make it a useful operational device in our modern world.

20.6 Big Data Jargon

A problem to traditional scientists is the jargon and numerous abbreviations applied by data scientists. A few examples will be given.

1. Data scientists themselves believe, that they are even more than 50% of their time spending on, what they call data cleaning. They tend to use jargon terms like e.g., data munging, a pejorative term, literally meaning changing the data to the extent, that they are entirely destructed. Mung is an abbreviation of mash until "no good". In Google Science Armand Ruiz, contributor to Infoworld even states, that most data scientists spend only 20% of their time on actual data analysis and 80% on cleaning and reorganizing huge amounts of data, which is, what he believes, a very inefficient data strategy (https://www.infoworld.com/article/3228245/data-science/the-80-20-data-science-dilemma.html).
2. Wikipedia, the free online encyclopedia gives examples of validations within the context of big data. They particularly include cross validations (not meaning second procedures, but, rather, the requirement of a second signal for each observation), and range validations (meaning validation is only approved if observations are within a defined max and min value), (https://en.wikipedia.org/wiki/Data_validation).

3. Many Big Data systems make use of Hadoop clusters. HDFS (Hadoop Distributing File Systems) distribute data through nodes (which may be computers or servers) in a cluster. Doug Cutting at Yahoo started Hadoop in 2015. He extended his prior work with the Nutch open soarce web crawler, where a crawler is here a system capable of systematically browsing the World Wide Web. To Hadoop even more worrisome than validation of data was distribution and storage of data.
4. Big data systems are particularly aiming at:
    1. User friendliness: data need not necessarily be saved in rows and columns (table-like), they should rather be saved like for example big text data, without a necessary structure.
    2. Scalibility: in the IT world meaning, that it can be made bigger without loss of properties.
5. A major disadvantage of the above points is, the likelihood of chaotic structures left, hardly capable of making contributions anymore to human understanding. They are called data lakes or, even more pejoratively, data sinks.

Traditional database uses SQL (Structured Query Language, used to communicate with data base). It is structured in the form of tables prior to storage. The jargon for this type of storage is "Scheme on right". With big data (using "NoSQL") the SQL structure needs to be realized afterwards, and prior to any further analysis. The jargon: "scheme on read". Big data require, in addition to the above traditional standards of validation, the process of Data verification, of which turning "schemes on read" will be an important element.

20.7 Discussion

Validation may be a semantic term. Yet it is, generally, agreed, that validation is the most important part of clinical studies, both small and big data studies, and that it currently demands more than half of the time spent on big data analysis (Xie C, Big data validation case study. Published by IEEE Computer Society, 2017, Doi 10.1109 BigDataService). In clinical research the term validation refers, according to the American FDA, to process design, process qualification, continuous process verification, and different types are implicated, like retrospective, prospective, concurrent validation, and re-validation. With diagnostic tests, which is commonly called the basis of clinical research, validation consists of accuracy, reproducibility, precision assessments. With clinical trial protocols validation consists of a clearly defined prior hypothesis, a valid design, explicit description of methods, and uniform data analysis.

Validating big data can, theoretically, be accomplished using all of the rules applied with small data, but this is very laborious, if not hardly possible. If big data consists of a pool of multiple small data, special checks are required, like publication bias, heterogeneity, robustness checks. Tentative alternatives for big data validation are occasionally given. In the above reference from Xie; multiple teams are appointed to validate fractions of data analyses. In the Hadoop framework (2014), an open-source framework to process and store big data (www.tutorialspoint.com), multiple standard computers with multiple relatively simple programs are applied for accomplishing big data validations.

The current chapter summarizes traditional validation tools for relatively small data, and, in addition, refers to important tentative tools especially designed for big data validation. We have to admit that many big data tools are commercial software, are very expensive, and have not been judged by Academia leave alone met by Academia standards.

References

Becker D, King T, Mcmullen B (2015) Big data, big data quality problem. Proceedings of IEEE international conference on bog data, pp 2264–3053.

Gao G, Xie C, Tao C (2016) Big data validation and quality assurance issues, challenges and needs. In: Proceedings of IEEE symposium on service oriented system engineering, Oxford, UK, pp 433–441.

Gassman J, Owens W, Kuntz T, Martin J, Amoroso W (1995) Data quality assurance, monitoring, and reporting. Control Clin Trials 16:104–136

Laranjeiro N, Soydemir S, Bernardino J (2015) A survey on data quality, classifying poor data. In: Proceedings of IEEE 21st Pacific Rim international symposium, pp 179–188.

Woodall P, Gao J, Parlikad A, Koronios A (2015) Classifying data quality problems in asset management. Springer Publications, Heidelberg

Index

T. J. Cleophas, A. H. Zwinderman, *Efficacy Analysis in Clinical Trials an Update*,
https://doi.org/10.1007/978-3-030-19918-0

The manufacturer's authorised representative in the EU is Springer Nature Customer Service Centre GmbH, Europaplatz 3, 69115 Heidelberg, Germany. If you have any concerns regarding our products, please contact ProductSafety@springernature.com

Printed and bound by CPI Group (UK) Ltd, Croydon, CR0 4YY
23/07/2026
02175017-0001